AF664958

COVID-19 PANDEMIC:
A Third Eye

AMITAV BANERJEE

BlueRose ONE .com
Stories Matter

First Published in March 2022

ISBN: 978-93-93388-69-8

BLUEROSE PUBLISHERS

www.BlueRoseONE.com

info@bluerosepublishers.com

+91 8882 898 898

Cover Design:

Aveek

Typographic Design:

Tanya Raj Upadhyay

Distributed by: BlueRose, Amazon, Flipkart

Preface

A few words on the origin of these columns would be in place. After an eventful and enriching professional career in the armed forces, the latter part of which was spent working as a field epidemiologist investigating outbreaks of communicable diseases in different terrains of the country, including tribal areas, I opted for a more quiet life. Towards this end, after prematurely hanging up my uniform, I took a teaching job in a medical school. This, while ideal for a sedate life, also sedated young energetic people who were compelled to attend lectures beyond their attention span.

Just when I was preparing for a second retirement and looking forward to rest my tired bones, I along with my students, while following the evolving pandemic and the responses globally, were woken up from the slumber. The chaos and anarchy resulting in equal measures by the impact of the virus and more often, due the responses in combating it were unparalleled in the history of public health.

Informal discussions with my students and colleagues brought out some fascinating patterns of the impact of the novel virus. I gave the tedious tasks of tabulating global data on the pandemic and correlating them with likely risk factors such as overweight proportion and median age of different countries to my students. What started out as a chore, soon gave way to excitement when we discerned a pattern suggesting that the pandemic was driven more by demographic and obesity profiles of different continents rather than any control measures which on the most part, were draconian and unprecedented in recent public health history.

These brainstorming sessions went beyond the confines of our institution. Often we got triggers from the "WhatsApp University" as well. The churning of ideas topping up the scattered sundry pieces accumulated through the years spent as a field epidemiologist which were lying, all jumbled up, and in disarray in the grey matter provided the material for serving this dish of potpourri.

These columns appeared in National Herald published from New Delhi and subsequently from Mumbai, from April to December 2021. Maj Gen V K Sinha, retired, introduced me to Uttam Sengupta, senior journalist, National Herald. Under their joint mentorship these columns took shape. My long time association with senior journalists like Umesh Isalkar of Times of India helped me grasp the nuances of writing for a target audience of laypersons.

As these column chronicling the pandemic rolled out, appreciation and criticisms, in equal measure, reflecting the polarization of views in this pandemic, provided insights for subsequent columns. For this I must specifically thank, Padmashree Dr Chandrakant Pandav who by his inspiring words, encouraged my writing. Others who provided valuable feedbacks are, Dr Sanjay Dabhade (who suggested the title), Dr Gautam Das, Dr Sthabir Dasgupta, Dr Sachin Atre, Dr Sarika Chaturvedi, Dr Jacob Puliyel, Mr Pallav Moitra, Dr Sanjay Rai, Maj Gen Y K Sharma, VSM, retired, Col S K Patra, retired, Dr Himadri Bal, Dr Sudhir Jadhav, Dr Hetal Rathod, Dr Kajal Shrivastava, Dr Swati Ghonge, Dr Khedkar, Mr Ashish Banerjee, and many colleagues. Often the columns received praise from Dr Bhagyashree Patil, Pro-Chancellor of Dr DY Patil Vidyapeeth, Pune. I got many a trigger from vibrant young minds, notably Aryan, Harsh, Uzair, Diptarka, Anushree and Arpan.

Dr Pranay Goel of Indian Institute of Science Education and Research, Pune, often triggered full columns by his insightful single liners.

I want to put on record the contribution of my research team, i.e. our residents consisting of Sweta, Biswajit, Kavita,

Sandeep, Vallari, Gracia, Prerna, Nirankush, Deepu, Johnson and Anil. They researched and verified the factual information for these columns.

I thank Professor Bhaskaran Raman, from Indian Institute of Technology, Bombay, for his sketches which speak more than words.

I owe a lot to two brilliant eye surgeons, Dr Akhil Bharadwaj and Dr Jeevan Kale, who managed the retinal detachment I developed during this period. Timely and skillful surgery and subsequent visual rehabilitation by their painstaking efforts helped me regain my vision enabling me to continue these columns without much interruption.

No person can claim to be a hero in the house. I am grateful to my close and extended family for tolerating my obsession with the same topic *ad nauseam*. My wife, Taposi, bore the brunt of this madness and deserves the highest praise. Others include Anubha, Ankan, Arundhati and Saurav. I feel the pain of Arundhati who lost her father in this pandemic.

I am sure there are many I have failed to acknowledge - my apologies to them.

Amitav Banerjee

Pune

26 January 2022

Contents

The Pandemic of Panic caused by overwhelming numbers, not lethality of the virus

Politics and commerce may have triumphed over science. India has had a vaccine for Tuberculosis for decades but with zero effectiveness on the Indian Population.

The pandemic of panic is reminiscent of a medieval era. Hasty decisions were taken giving and maintaining an illusion of control. These crude and clumsy measures have fractured society and will have long term economic impact.

How the world arrived at this predicament? As the pandemic originated in Wuhan in Hubei district, China, this country became the pacesetter in this marathon. Being the *bête-noire* of most nations whatever drastic measures China implemented was roundly criticised by the Western media and even the WHO. The WHO representative remarked that the lockdown of Hubei district in China, of 56 million people was unprecedented in public health history and certainly not approved by the WHO. Western media and legal experts dubbed China's actions as 'harsh,' 'severe,' 'extreme' and 'controversial,' unlikely to control the virus. They stressed on the darker side of lockdown, being unscientific and authoritarian.

Who would have imagined that China had effectively done its role as pacesetter and nation after nation including democracies will outdo China in implementing these draconian measures. Concerns about the dark side and authoritarianism of such harsh measures seemed to have been forgotten. The experts advocated this to 'flatten the curve' and 'break the chain of transmission' some of the jargons thrown up as the pandemic progressed relentlessly.

The cross country marathon lost the way early due to misleading cues. The lethality of the virus was grossly overestimated in the early days as it was calculated from hospital admitted cases comprising mostly the elderly. The median age of fatal cases in Italy in early days of the pandemic was 80 years. The Lancet in March 2020 suggested that the case fatality rate can be as high as 20%. Subsequent studies including serosurveys refined the infection fatality rate to as low as 0.27% as most infections are asymptomatic and mild cases in the community are only detected by antibody levels during population surveys. However, first impressions last. The early impression of high lethality continues to provoke panic among the masses to this day. This is aggravated by reports of lack of hospital beds and oxygen presently faced by our country in the unprecedented and unexpected second wave. In fact according to the third round of national level serosurvey carried out by the ICMR, the infection fatality rate can be roughly estimated to be 0.05% in our country.

In the second wave, we were overwhelmed by numbers and not by the lethality of the virus alone. The pandemic exposed cracks in our public health infrastructure and inequitable distribution of health services. Corporate model of health system focused in big cities are not geared to face public health emergencies like pandemics. Even in normal times, the out-of-pocket expenditure for health services drives many poor families below the poverty line. Because of this mismatch of supply and demand, we had an acute emergency on our hands but not squarely due to covid. The common man faced the grim situation of lack of adequate medical care what the poor and marginalized have been facing for years.

The scientific community too lost the plot early, sometimes by omission and sometimes, regrettably, by commission. Prediction models based on computer simulation instead of epidemiological surveillance predicted doomsday. These caused shock and awe. More serious are doubts concerning scientific integrity. An editorial in the British Medical Journal

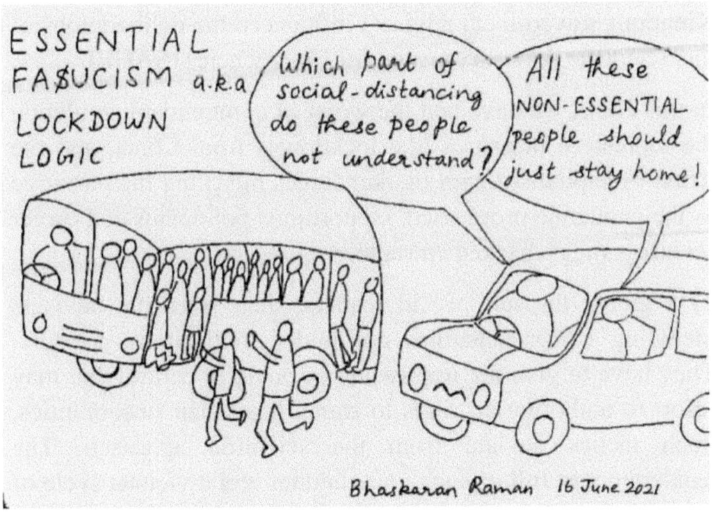
ESSENTIAL FA$UCISM a.k.a LOCKDOWN LOGIC
Which part of social-distancing do these people not understand?
All these NON-ESSENTIAL people should just stay home!
Bhaskaran Raman 16 June 2021

(BMJ) by K Abbasi, titled, 'Covid-19, Politicisation, Corruption, and Suppression of Science,' raises concerns about the science, or rather, the lack of it during the pandemic. It puts forth, rather candidly, that science was being suppressed by politicians, and governments ostensibly in the public interest. Making the issue murkier are conflicts of interest of academics, researchers and commercial lobbies.

The scientific debate gave way to polarization with eminent scientists on both sides of the divide on issues of Covid-19 control. The vast majority were silent fearing professional repercussions. Politics and commercial interests replaced science driving policy. The New Indian Express on 20 September 2020 alleged that the Indian Council of Medical Research (ICMR), under political influence, firewalled crucial data of serosurvey conducted to assess the spread of Covid-19 spread. Such reports erode public trust in scientists.

As reported in the BMJ editorial, even in developed countries, politics meddled with scientific reports. Political appointees within the US Department of Health demanded to review and revise scientific statements related to Covid-19 published by the Centre of Disease Control and Prevention. In the United

Kingdom, government advisers influenced the deliberations of the Scientific Advisory Group for Emergencies (SAGE).

In this crisis, we have had the worst of communism emulating the repressive measures like lockdowns from China, and the worst of capitalism with market forces hijacking the narrative as the pandemic progressed. Opportunist politicians and career scientists piggy-backed en route.

In a global disaster, world leaders, their scientific advisers including career scientists are under tremendous pressure. They have to give the impression of being in control and may resort to authoritarian ways to camouflage their uncertainties. Such tactics deviate from the scientific approach. The pandemic was full of such uncertainties and a vicious cycle of repression set in when the authorities and their advisers were faced with rising case numbers or dissenting views.

The tendency was to blame the people for not observing appropriate precautions, most of which like social distancing are difficult in densely populated countries. There was even a joke circulating that if all Indians were to maintain social distancing, we will enter neighbouring countries! And most of these non-pharmacological interventions were based on computer simulations which considered humans as inert units and not as social beings who cannot live in a bubble insulated from their environment. Attempts to do so cause greater harm to health by way of psychological disorders.

The collateral damage to children who are losing on schooling and social development was also considerable. And of course people lost livelihoods, which translate in loss of lives.

The arrival of the vaccine also brought its sets of dilemmas. The world medical consensus seemed to go for a win against corona, i.e. eradication of the disease. This is unprecedented in public health history. The vaccines had hit the ground running. The effectiveness data on population level was too early to predict. Going all out for mass vaccination with uncertain input on effectiveness was a big gambit. We have a vaccine against tuberculosis for decades which has zero effectiveness in preventing tuberculosis in the Indian population. Moreover, there are concerns that haphazard and incomplete vaccination of the population can trigger mutant strains. All these concerns, like almost anything concerning the novel coronavirus, needed more detailed research.

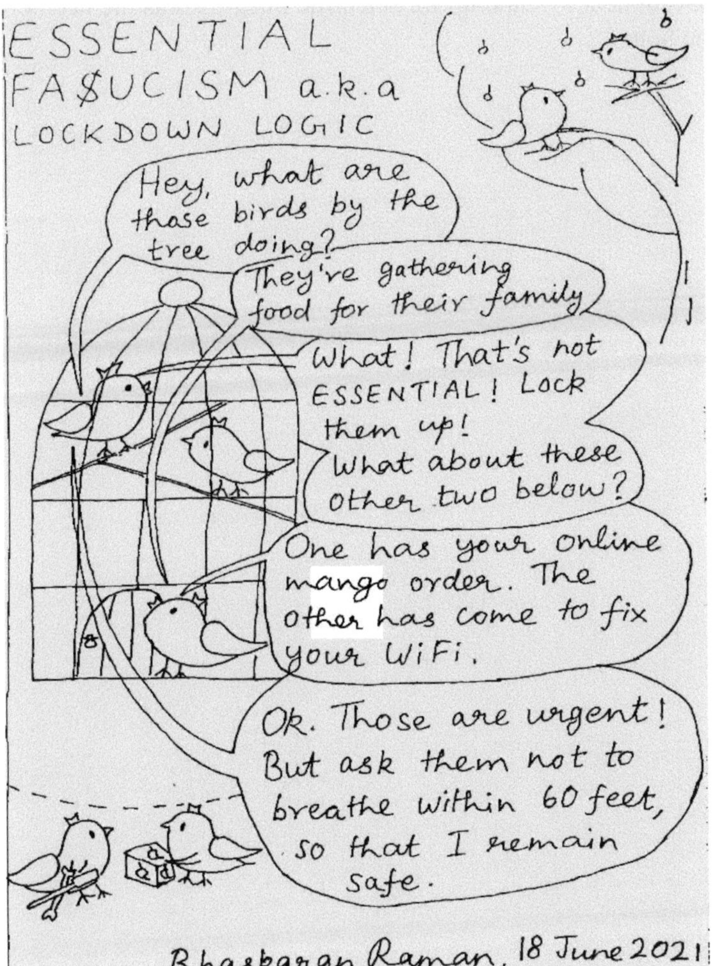

A scientific temperament should be able to contemplate diverse opinions with detachment and equipoise and subject them to proper scientific enquiry. Unfortunately, such an approach was lacking. Any opinion contrary to the consensus was brushed under the carpet if not censored. There was opacity and obfuscation instead of transparency. Moral courage among our scientists in advisory positions to the government to stand up for scientific integrity was the need of the hour.

Second Thoughts on Mass Vaccination.

Vaccination without monitoring, surveillance and countrywide serosurvey is not helpful; it is like running a superfast train on old rickety tracks. The vaccine is a powerful weapon and needs to be deployed strategically

Elon Musk had famously remarked that he and his family would not take the Covid-19 vaccine. Coming from a celebrity multibillionaire and entrepreneur such a statement is likely to promote vaccine hesitancy among many. On the other hand, the unprecedented second wave with reports of scarcity of oxygen and hospital beds led to desperation among the masses who believed that mass vaccination will halt the pandemic in its tracks. This was evident from the crowds at the vaccination centres and frequent crashing of the CoWIN application, the online site for registration. Both extreme positions, outright rejection of vaccine by public figures on one hand, and on the other, craze to get vaccinated by the masses, can adversely affect fight against any pandemic.

Vaccine is a strong and powerful weapon against the novel coronavirus. A marvel of modern precision and genomic technology. And like all strong weapons, it should neither be withheld nor used indiscriminately but should be deployed strategically to derive maximum benefit in a cost-effective way. The generals of the war against the pandemic should be conversant with the benefits as well as the hazards of this artillery, the vaccine.

"Therefore those who are not thoroughly aware of the disadvantages in the use of arms cannot be thoroughly aware of the advantages in the use of arms." Sun Tzu [Art of War].

Sun Tzu, ironically, was a Chinese General around 500 BC whose treatise The Art of War influences military thinking and strategy to this day. Might as well apply his strategy to combat a virus which originated in his homeland, China!

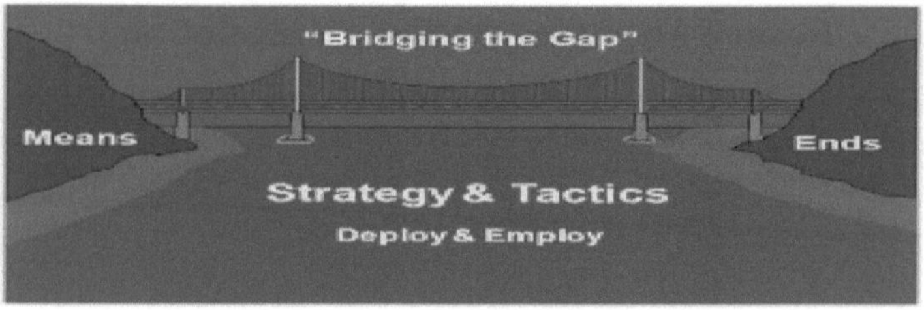

Like a good general, we should have preserved our ammunition, the vaccine. A good military commander, surveys the lay of the land before deploying his heavy ammunition, the artillery. Using this analogy, we should have been guided by our logistics and epidemiological data to prioritise vaccination rather than opening vaccine for all during early stages of the pandemic. Fighting on all fronts simultaneously drains the army of health workers and resources and, with a leaky vaccine, hardly has an impact given our large population.

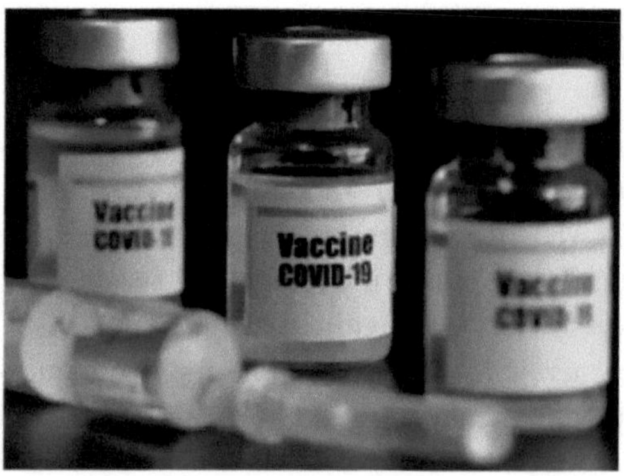

Regrettably, nobody paid heed to these ground realities, in spite of occasional sane counsel by national experts. Dr N K Arora, Head, Operations Research Group at Indian Council of Medical Research (ICMR), wrote an opinion piece dated April 12, 2021, in the Times of India, titled, 'Opening up vaccines for younger adults right now will be a gamble with lives.' He went on to explain the logistic challenges and the science behind this strategy. He stated that it would have made perfect sense to vaccinate all adults if we lived in an utopia with infinite resources. However, the reality was that we were in the midst of a raging pandemic with finite supplies of vaccines. The aim was to reduce deaths and hospitalization from the infection. There was limited evidence that current vaccine can interrupt transmission. Young adults without co-morbidites rarely landed up in hospital or died from the infection. So vaccinating young adults will not be cost effective. What needed to be done was to prevent deaths the majority of which occured in the older age groups. Dr Arora also warned about the possibility of emergence of mutant strains as a result of mass and indiscriminate vaccination campaigns.

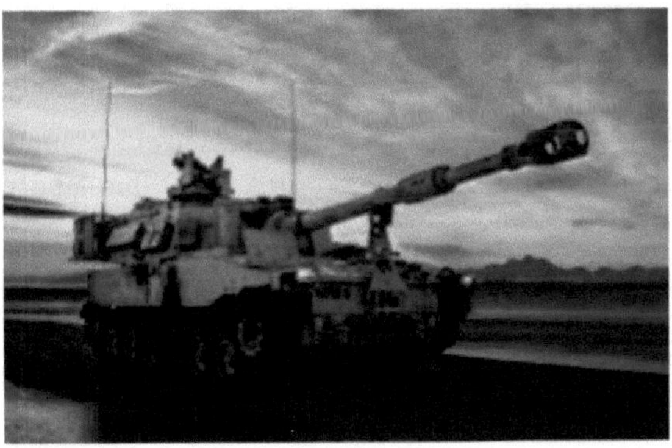

Made perfect sense. However subsequent events indicate little heed was being paid to logic and science in this pandemic. Within a couple of weeks of this recommendation, many state governments announced vaccination of all adults over 18 years, some even declaring it free. Playing to the gallery. A barely concealed example of populist demagogy. Any opposition to this ostensibly welfare measure was labelled as '"vaccine hesitancy'..." Bureaucrats and scientific advisers to the government were afraid to be stigmatized thus, and fearing repercussions, tended to remain silent. Group think prevailed in this environment and all felt secure on the bandwagon. Ironically, later in the pandemic, even Dr N K Arora overruled the reservations of the National Technical Advisory of Government of India (NTAGI) regarding vaccination for children! A perfect example of an opportunistic career scientist!

Unfortunately, remarkable scientific progress like precision medicine and genomics which steered vaccine developments in record time deprived the proponents of these and the public of common sense. It got worse when market forces entered the picture. Woody Allen says in Annie Hall, '"...that's the thing with intellectuals, they can be absolutely brilliant, but still have no idea what is going on.'"

Due to the vicious pace of the second wave and subsequently the latest variant, Omicron, which ran amuck in our country, it became clear that mass vaccination of the population will not catch up with the pace of natural infections among our population. And most of these infections were asymptomatic or mild, particularly with Omicron. Against this landscape, it was wasteful use of resources to go for mass scale population vaccination in our country for a disease which had very low consequences for the young and healthy.

According to the third round of National Level Serosurvey, about 21% of our population had already encountered the virus during the first wave. Given the speed of spread of the second wave and its scale, it is very likely that another 30-50% of the population got infected before the vaccine reached them. At the end of the second wave about 50-70% of our population reached some level of population immunity due to natural infection as revealed by serosurveys. There is no scientific logic to vaccinate those who have recovered from natural infection whatsoever the '"experts'" say based on conjectures and not on real world data or principles of immunology.

There are other issues related to mass vaccination which can lead to vaccine hesitancy among the masses. If millions are vaccinated at fast pace with limited resources for monitoring and surveillance of adverse events following vaccination, there are likely to be some adverse events, and deaths which may be purely coincidental and not related to the vaccines. Even so, common perception would attribute it to the vaccine leading to vaccine hesitancy. This will be a setback which would make it difficult to administer vaccine to even the vulnerable.

To practice and follow hard science, we should have gone for country wide serosurveys once the second wave was over for estimating the population level immunity. We should have refrained from vaccinating those with antibodies and also those who have had a positive RT-PCR report in the past. This would have saved a lot of vaccines and resources which could have been focused on those who really needed the vaccine such as health care workers, front line workers, the elderly and people with obesity and co-morbidities. To continue the science we could have followed large cohorts who had recovered from past infections to see whether they got re-infected. We could have revised our vaccination policy guided by science if we did find an appreciable number of re-infections which were serious enough.

The pace in the pandemic was like running a marathon at the speed of a sprint. Everything from the diagnostic test on which so many policy decisions were taken, lockdowns, most treatment regimes, and the vaccines developed at warp speed, were on emergency use authorization modes unprecedented in the history of public health.

The medical consensus has reached the last lap of this marathon, or thinks it has, the finishing line being eradication. Politicians and the public alike think that the vaccines will eradicate the coronavirus. But history of public health does not support this hope. Only one disease, smallpox could be eradicated more than hundred and fifty years after arrival of its vaccine. It was a disease which required no sophisticated diagnostic test, did not have subclinical and asymptomatic infections, cases could be identified and isolated even by the common people and the smallpox virus did not infect animals. None of these criteria applies to the coronavirus.

Given these realities, it is time to take a pause in this marathon, and revise our strategy based on science and common sense and not based on tunnel visions of laboratory scientists, however brilliant, and political expediencies.

Towards this end, an open letter from top scientists in the country, published on 29 April asked the government for access to databases on Covid-19 testing. Data captured by government agencies like the ICMR can drive evidence based public health policy. Data on age, location, health and vaccination status of everyone who submits a sample for Covid-19 test should be made easily accessible. Such data can help prioritize groups for vaccination, help us understand the role of concurrent illnesses, and enable evaluation of the efficacy of vaccines.

What explains the death of relatively young Indians to Covid-19?

Sufficient data and studies are not there to draw firm conclusions. But a large section of the young are obese and many of them in both rural and urban areas are unaware they are diabetic.

One of the most dreadful impressions during the second wave of this pandemic was that, this time around, the virus was mostly attacking younger people. Fuel to fire was fed by vivid descriptions of young patients succumbing to the infection, or more disturbingly, narration of serious complications in children. So much so, the medical consensus seemed to predict that the third wave will hit the paediatric age group. This impression gained ground by inputs from well meaning clinicians working round the clock. Media reports fuelled the panic in the population.

The fascinating discipline of epidemiology can be compared to chess. The epidemiologist sees the whole board. As doctors, we all start with clinical medicine and the majority continue in this stream. Few choose epidemiology and public health, the less glamorous, the somewhat abstract discipline. Even during pandemics eminent clinicians are sought for their views being well known public figures.

The transformation from clinical medicine to epidemiology is akin to a chess player evolving to masters' level. In pandemics, clinicians and epidemiologists will have different perspectives. Clinicians contributed immensely in the crises, some even with their lives. As a result, treatment regimes got refined, and case fatality rates came down considerably. However, they are not ideally positioned to see the dynamics of pandemics in the population.

There was no marked difference in the age profiles of people affected with Covid-19 in the second wave compared to the first. This was stated in an official briefing around end of April

2021, by Dr V K Paul, a paediatrician, member of Niti Ayog and Dr Balram Bhargava, Director General of Indian Council of Medical Research (ICMR). They elaborated that in the second wave 32% of the cases were below 30 years, as compared to 31% in the first. The average age of patients in the second wave was 49 years compared to 50 in the previous year. In the first wave there was 4.2% of patients between 0 to 19 years, in the second it was 5.8%; while the 20-40 years bracket comprises 25% of the case load in the second compared to 23% in the first wave..

Why the panic, including an amateurish editorial in Lancet? The speed, spike and bounce of the second wave took everyone by surprise. Let us analyse our strengths and weakness, which will help us predict how we are going to fare in future pandemics.

Like most Asian and African countries we have a demographic advantage. We have a broad base of young adults and children to cushion the full impact of mild to moderate pandemics. Sweden which did not close schools during the pandemic supports this proposition. In spite of schools being open throughout, there was no excess morbidity or mortality among the Swedish school children or their school staff.

Comparison of overweight prevalence based on Body Mass Index (BMI) show that countries in the West have overweight prevalence around 60% compared to around 20% in the Asian and African Countries. Age and obesity drove mortality rates from corona virus 10 to 20 times higher in the developed world compared to developing countries.

Two outlier countries provide clue to this question with interesting contrasts.

Japan has the highest age profile, but their obesity profile is one-third of the West. Their mortality from Covid-19 was almost 15 times less than the Western countries. The strongest piece in Japan appeared to be overall good health as evidenced by low BMI of the population.

The other outlier country was Brazil, which holds important lessons for India. It had lower age profile but obesity profile was similar to the West. Like India it is a rapidly developing economy with change in lifestyle, physical activity and diet. The mortality from Covid-19 in Brazil exceeded that in many Western countries. Obesity proved to be a greater driver of lethality than age.

Will future pandemics affect the young? While overall we have a lean population, there is a tendency for the recently affluent population to adopt sedentary lifestyles, fast food, alcohol and smoking. Moreover, due to genetic handicap, Indians are more prone to diabetes and diseases of coronary heart disease a decade or two earlier than their Caucasian counterpart.

What is the way forward? We have to beef up the public health infrastructure equitably, and address the lifestyle changes among the newly affluent. A number of studies in our field practice areas brought out these incipient trends among the youth and young adults

We found the younger generation four times more likely to be deficient in Vitamin D compared to the older generation. Diabetes was fairly prevalent in our rural and urban population, and more than half younger diabetics in the 35 to 45 years age group were not aware of their diabetes status. Risk factors of non-communicable diseases were prevalent both among urban and rural youth and young people.

Childhood malnutrition remains quite high as brought out in studies by our postgraduates and faculty.

We lose about 2000 under five children every day due to preventable diseases against a background of child malnutrition. Loss of livelihoods and interruption of child community nutrition programs at the community level will increase child malnutrition and child deaths. While pandemics may be mild on the child with normal nutrition, severe malnutrition in children may make them vulnerable.

If we do not address these concerns, we may have future pandemics in which young people and children will bear the brunt, not due to lack of vaccination, as the present amateurish consensus seems to suggest, but as a result of not addressing the modifiable risk factors.

If like an amateur strategist we look only at the major piece the new queen, the vaccine, we may be left holding the queen but losing the game.

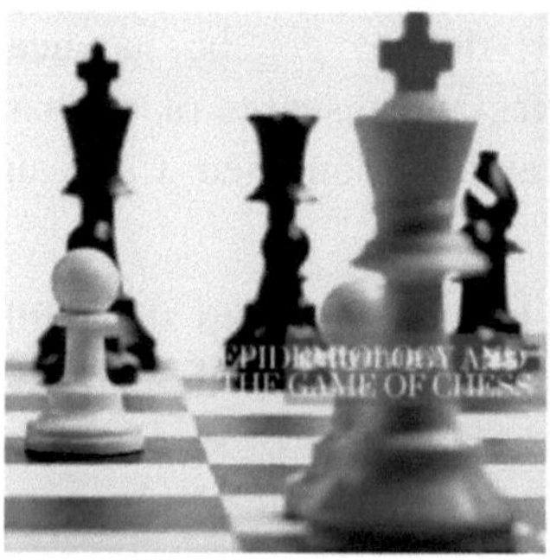

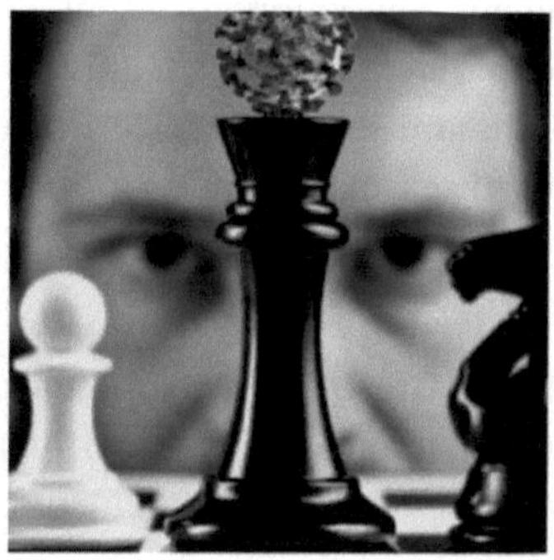

What evolutionary biology tells us about coronavirus mutants?

Most mutations have no impact on virulence or infectivity. Viruses which kill also perish with the host. Strains that survive are not lethal.

A former Chief Minister of an Indian State got into trouble when he remarked, '"Coronavirus also has a right to live!"' He was trolled heavily on social media.

David Deutsch in his provocative book, '"The Beginning of Infinity,"' states that when we seek explanations, we lean towards anthropocentrism, explaining things parochially from the human perspective. To balance this is anti-anthropocentrism epitomized by '"The Principle of Mediocrity,"' which assumes that there is nothing significant about humans in the cosmic scheme of things.

One does not know whether the former Chief Minister had read this book. Politicians have little time for reading. But he had a point, perhaps unknowingly.

The pandemic, driven by anthropocentrism, became protracted. What promised to be a sprint turned out to be a marathon. Did we take the right path? And being in sprint mode, did we go too far in the wrong direction in this cross country race? Did chasing the virus at all costs turned into a prestige issue for world governments and their scientific advisers, an extreme form of anthropocentricism?

The strategy of lockdowns, physical distancing and school closures, which became a recurrent strategy, was based on a computer simulation project on control of influenza pandemics by a high school student, daughter of an American scientist. Similarly, studies on hamsters on benefit of masks guided mask mandate. Subsequently, a Danish randomized trial on masks and later a study from Bangladesh, were inconclusive.

However, the guidelines regarding mask, continued to get more stringent, from single mask to double-mask stage.

The one single theme in the pandemic was "'Fear is the Key.'" Citizens of almost all countries, including major democracies, complied with measures which deprived them of their fundamental rights, driven by the common denominator of panic. A major contributor to the pandemic of panic were the draconian measures which has no precedence in the history of public health.

Projecting number of cases and deaths of one disease out of context can easily generate panic in the population. This has never been done for any disease ever. This resulted in mass obsessive compulsive disorder around one disease. Everything about the novel disease assumed larger than life dimensions. In the initial days it was transmission from surfaces, which was later discarded, thankfully. Later, there were reports that air borne small particles or nuclei can be carried up to ten meters. Cause for further panic. Conveniently overlooking that within this radius there may be millions of microbes surrounding us, in addition to the billions within us. The latest agenda for mass hysteria are media reports of mutant variants of the novel coronavirus. Popular perception would be that mutants generate monsters. Evolutionary biology tells us otherwise.

Coming back to the "'faux pas'" of the former chief minister, viruses also have a right to live. Whether we like it or not, nature grants them a fair chance. To survive, they follow nature's way of adaptation – Darwin's Law.

These adaptations are by way of mutations, natural phenomena, not new, due to errors during replication, and occasionally due to selection pressure. According to principles of successful parasitism, this adaptation is beneficial to both the virus and humans. Errors that make the virus fittest for survival propagate while others lose out due to natural selection.

Lethal or virulent strains do not go far. Viruses which kill perish with the host leading to a dead end infection. Lesser virulent ones which do not kill but cause symptoms will also phase out because of of self- isolation.

The mutant strains, which will survive and go far, will be the less virulent strains which do not kill the host, produce very mild symptoms or none at all. People infected with such mild variants will mix with others and transmit widely. High contagiousness does not translate to high virulence. Such strains promote population immunity with minimum casualties.

How does mutation take place? The novel coronavirus SARS-CoV-2 is a RNA virus, which has about 30, 000 base pairs of nitrogen compounds, about 3000 to 4000 are in the spike protein. These base pairs can be considered as the building bricks of the virus. Addition, deletion or changes in sequence within these building bricks lead to mutation.

What can be the implications of mutation? There are a number of possibilities. Most mutations have no impact on virulence or infectivity. They are used as fingerprints for tracing the path of outbreaks. Some mutations will become less virulent but more infective, with better chances of survival and propagation by law of natural selection. And rarely, they may become more virulent, such outliers would also lose the evolutionary race.

The following are the concerns related to mutation. Will vaccine work? Will immunity obtained after recovery from natural infection work? Will RT-PCR detect the mutant variants?

Antibodies and immune cells generated by natural infections or vaccination act on some of the building blocks known as epitopes. As mentioned the novel coronavirus has about 30,000 base pairs or building blocks of nitrogen compounds. During mutations only a few of the building blocks undergo change. So antibodies and immune cells primed against the whole virus as on recovery from natural infection or immunization by a vaccine derived from the whole virus have very good chance of neutralizing these variants.

Some vaccines target only the spike protein or more specifically few of the building blocks in them. These targets are known as epitopes, out of 3000-4000 of these base pairs in the spike protein. If mutation occurs in an epitope in the spike protein there is slightly more chance of antibodies and immune cells hitting a blank on a mutated epitope. However, as many epitopes are involved in the process, such vaccines will also confer some protection against the mutants. The RT-PCR tests which target a number of epitopes should also detect variants.

It should also be somewhat reassuring that due to principles of evolutionary biology, mutants which will dominate at the population level in the long run will be less virulent. This is the way of all pandemics. Over time they become seasonal minor illnesses. The concept is summed up in a dialogue from a popular Hindi Movie Agneepath, *'"Apna ussool kehta hai ... jab dushman ki umar badh jaaye toh usse dosti karlo ... apni umar badh jaati hai'" translated, '"My principle is...when the life of your enemy increases then befriend him...it increases your life also.'"*

[Author's note: Many technical concepts and terms have been oversimplified for better understanding of a larger audience]

Government jumped several red lights dealing with Covid.

The pandemic of Covid-19 led to a cascade of knee-jerk draconian measures by most countries of the world. The panic permeated the psyche of populations rendering them compliant to virtual house arrest. In this chaos and anarchy, almost all the ethical principles such as equity, beneficence, non-maleficence and autonomy were breached.

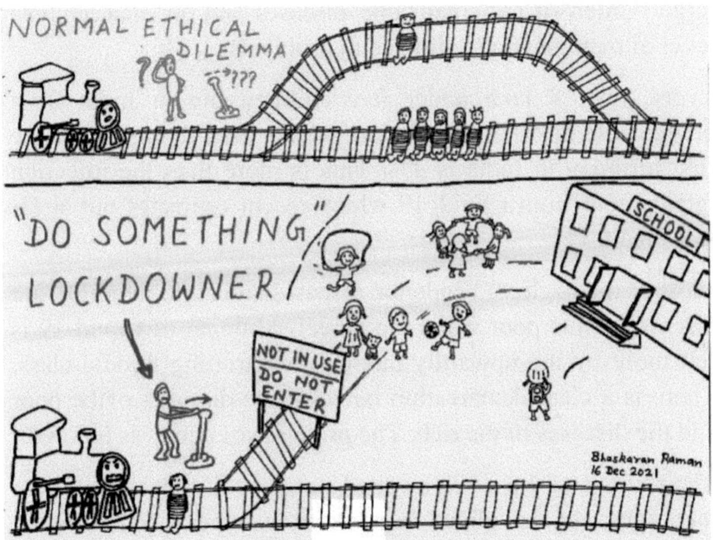

Covid-19 brought to focus that we have forgotten the lessons in Social Medicine painstakingly learned after the scientific world realized some of the limitations of the dogma of the '"Germ Theory of Disease"' following the discoveries of Robert Koch and Louis Pasteur in the nineteenth century. After the initial euphoria, it was realized that besides bacteria and viruses, there are social offshoots of infectious diseases. Diseases have social causes, social pathologies and social consequences. The road to social welfare consists of ethical red lights as safeguards from collateral harm. In this pandemic, all the red lights of ethics, i.e. Equity, Beneficence, Non Maleficence and Autonomy were ignored.

Equity

Equity or justice means that each person's interest should count equally. This by logic should also imply that all diseased persons irrespective of the diagnosis should have equal and easy access to health services. Each disease which is a public health problem should get equal attention. In India, we have a large burden of communicable diseases and an unacceptable level of maternal and child health problems.

Every year, 8 lakh under five children die in India from preventable diseases. The risk of a new born dying before the first birthday in India is 3%. This is more than the infection fatality rate from Covid- 19 which recent estimates put at far less than 0.1%.

Most of the neglected endemic diseases and child mortality are diseases of the poor while the perceived threat of Covid-19 is felt more by the upwardly mobile globetrotting middle class. There is a clear demarcation between the diseases of the poor and the diseases of the rich. The principle of equity is ignored.

The roll out of the much awaited vaccines further reveal these inequities. At the global level rich countries had unlimited vaccine supplies, while the poor countries struggled to procure adequate supplies. Within the country, there is urban rural divide in access to vaccines. There were reports of people from cities going to villages to get vaccinated depriving the uninformed rural residents of access to the vaccine.

Beneficence and Non-malfeasance

The ethical principle of beneficence implies that people should benefit from any intervention and risk benefit ratio should be acceptable. In this crises, lockdown was one of the greatest population level interventions. For the poor, the risk of fatality from contracting Covid-19 was far less than the risk of fatality from any of the other diseases of poverty which are endemic in India. Lockdowns pushed people to extreme poverty and misery. Child malnutrition and child deaths rose exponentially; no fancy models from overrated foreign universities were needed to predict this.

Non-malfeasance means do no harm. This is an important ethical principle of any intervention. The greatest harm in the lockdown with hardly any benefit was imposed on the marginalized section of the population.

According to the latest census, more than 6.4 crores of Indian population stays in slums. This is almost equal to the population of UK or France. Anyone who has visited a slum in India will know that social distancing or frequent hand-washing is just not possible for these marginalized people. Most of them share common community toilets with scant water and hand-washing facilities. Cooped up 24 hours in crowded living conditions would be the ideal situation for spread of respiratory infections besides other communicable diseases.

A feature in New York Times, dated 26 May 2021, reveals how the Center of Disease Control (CDC), USA misinterpreted a scientific paper to conclude that risk of Covid transmission outdoors is 10%. This led to advice to stay indoors and wearing of mask when stepping outdoors. Subsequently, one of the authors of the paper tweeted that risk of outdoor transmission was less than 0.1% and not 10% as reported by CDC, which overestimated the risk of outdoor transmission hundred fold! This fundamental error led to restriction of outdoor activities worldwide, and caller tunes urging us not to step outdoors, the American CDC being the bellwether for global mandates on Covid-19.

The co-author of the misinterpreted paper, Nooshin Razani further tweeted, "'…People should spend more time outdoors to enjoy nature and be active. Being outdoors is essentially the best ventilation one could ever imagine, as particles have the space to infinitely dilute, disperse, and eventually essentially disappear.'" In a subsequent interview she mentioned that the outdoors is the best resource and we should find ways to undertake most activities outdoors. In spite of this clarification by one of the authors of the paper on which the CDC based its recommendations to stay indoors, the august body and global consensus continue to treat outdoor activities as a major risk.

Had CDC followed the science correctly, it would not have continued to recommend restriction of outdoor activities and businesses. The cascade effect made other countries to follow suit and shut down all outdoor activities and businesses whenever there were surge in cases. This led to severe economic hardships particularly in developing countries where most people in the unorganized sector work outdoors.

The irony is that in developing countries, poor workers were pushed indoors in their crowded living conditions where they were more exposed to infections and to add insult to injury lost their livelihoods most of which are pursued in safer outdoor environments. These included hawkers, small traders on the roadside, open street food restaurant owners and so on. If we had followed the science, we could have ensured interruption of transmission which occurs predominantly indoors and also preserved livelihoods which depend on outdoor work.

Autonomy or informed choice.

The greatest lockdown in the world was announced, with good intentions, at a notice of four hours. Economists, social scientists and others were not given an opportunity in the public forum to voice their concerns. There was no public debate of the pros and cons of this draconian measure on such a large scale. Hundreds of lives and livelihoods continued to be at stake and vulnerable to the ravages of unemployment, hunger and starvation deaths. The Epidemic Disease Act 1897 from the colonial times enacted to fight the plague was enforced giving enormous powers to the state and suspension of many basic human rights. This was used to tackle a 21st century disease which should have been addressed by science and evidence rather than converting most countries into police states.

These ethical oversights need to be deliberated so that future pandemics do not evoke such clumsy and crude responses with the remedy worse than the problem.

Covid-19 –Data suggests there is a strong case for reopening schools.

Data suggests that there is a strong case for reopening schools. While more children indeed got infected in the second wave, it was more due to entire families getting infected. Data indicate Covid-19 rarely killed children.

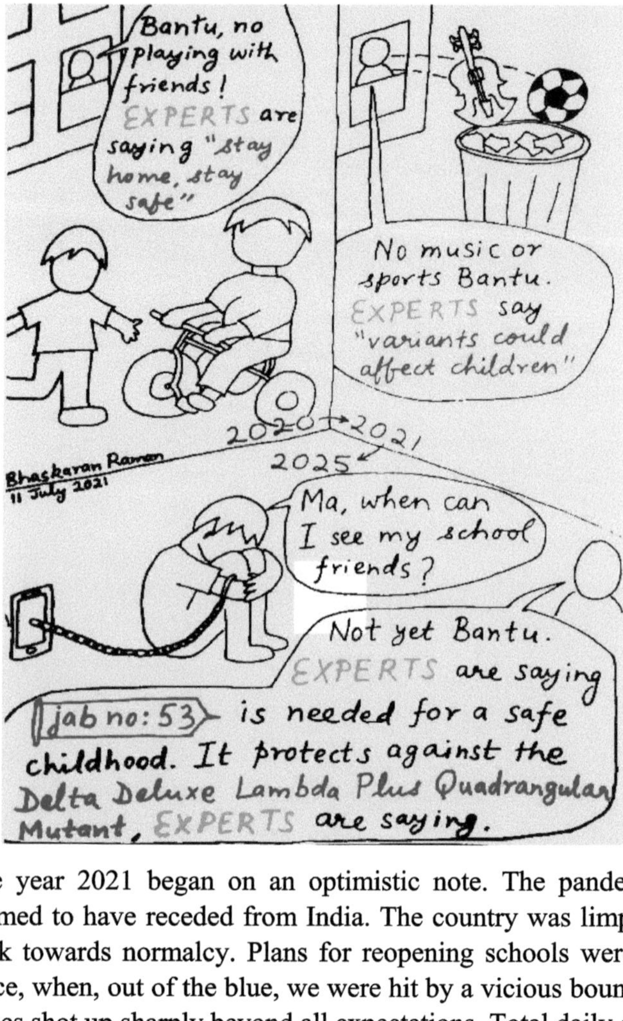
Bantu, no playing with friends! EXPERTS are saying "stay home, stay safe"
No music or sports Bantu. EXPERTS say "variants could affect children"
2020→2021
2025
Bhaskaran Raman
11 July 2021
Ma, when can I see my school friends?
Not yet Bantu. EXPERTS are saying
jab no: 53
is needed for a safe childhood. It protects against the Delta Deluxe Lambda Plus Quadrangular Mutant, EXPERTS are saying.

The year 2021 began on an optimistic note. The pandemic seemed to have receded from India. The country was limping back towards normalcy. Plans for reopening schools were in place, when, out of the blue, we were hit by a vicious bouncer. Cases shot up sharply beyond all expectations. Total daily case count at the peak around first week of May 2021 was four times higher than the first wave. Hospitals were overwhelmed. There were crises of beds and oxygen. The impact this time was also felt in the rural areas which had inadequate health infrastructure. Covid-19 patients from the villages travelled to urban areas to seek treatment adding to the crises.

Thankfully, the crises waned as sharply as it had escalated. Various reasons were put forward for the unexpected second wave including mutants with higher virulence and transmissibility. While mutations occurred, it does not fully explain the equally sharp fall of the curve.

Waxing and waning of transmission in a pandemic is a natural phenomenon irrespective of the '"illusion of control"' by humans. For the first time in recent public health history we tried to control the course of the pandemic by human interventions. Like the '"illusion of control"' we also were lulled by the '"illusion of success"' when the first wave receded. We were jolted out of this complacency by the sudden and sharp second wave. This should make us realize that lockdowns cannot prevent transmission; it can only postpone it, only to bounce back with interest.

In the second wave too, cases came down sharply not much due to human intervention but because the virus, possibly a more contagious variant, ran through most of the vulnerable people along with simultaneous development of herd immunity acting as a speed breaker. Vaccination had reached less than 10% of the large Indian population and cannot account for the abrupt fall. Moreover, at the height of a pandemic, vaccination has no impact as natural infections run through the population at faster pace. The fall cannot be attributed to lockdowns either as during the first wave the cases kept increasing even after imposing restrictive measures. Maharashtra had the highest duration and highest number of lockdowns as well as high number of cases.

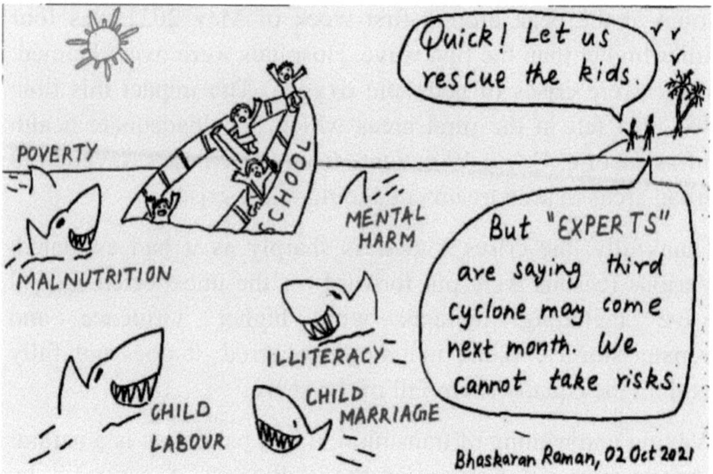
Quick! Let us rescue the kids.
But "EXPERTS" are saying third cyclone may come next month. We cannot take risks.
POVERTY
SCHOOL
MENTAL HARM
MALNUTRITION
ILLITERACY
CHILD LABOUR
CHILD MARRIAGE
Bhaskaran Raman, 02 Oct 2021

Whatever the reasons there were many concerns even as the second wave seems to be receding. Foremost was the fear that the third wave will be harsh on children. This was based on the premise that as the adult population gets vaccinated the virus will continue to circulate in children. Besides, hospitals during the second wave saw more paediatric admissions. This was not due to children being more vulnerable this time but due to rise in absolute numbers across all age groups. Understandably the perspective of clinicians was that in subsequent waves the impact would be felt mostly by children. However, hard data did not support these assumptions. Among the admitted cases, the proportion of children 0-18 years was between 2-5% in both the first and second waves. Data mining at global level indicated that children had negligible chances of severe disease and death compared to adults.

In a paper published in Public Health, UK, researchers analysed pooled data from seven countries which had faced the fury of the pandemic. They calculated child mortality from Covid-19 and compared it with deaths from other causes in children during the study period.

During the three months study period, there were 44 deaths in children among 42, 846 confirmed cases of Covid-19, giving a case fatality rate of 0.1%. For every detected case, there are 20-30 undetected cases, which would put the infection fatality rate in the age group 0-18 years below 0.005%. In the same period, the authors found 13, 200 deaths from other causes, most frequent being 1056 deaths due to accidents, 308 from lower respiratory diseases and 107 from influenza. Covid-19 in children contributed only 0.33% of all deaths.

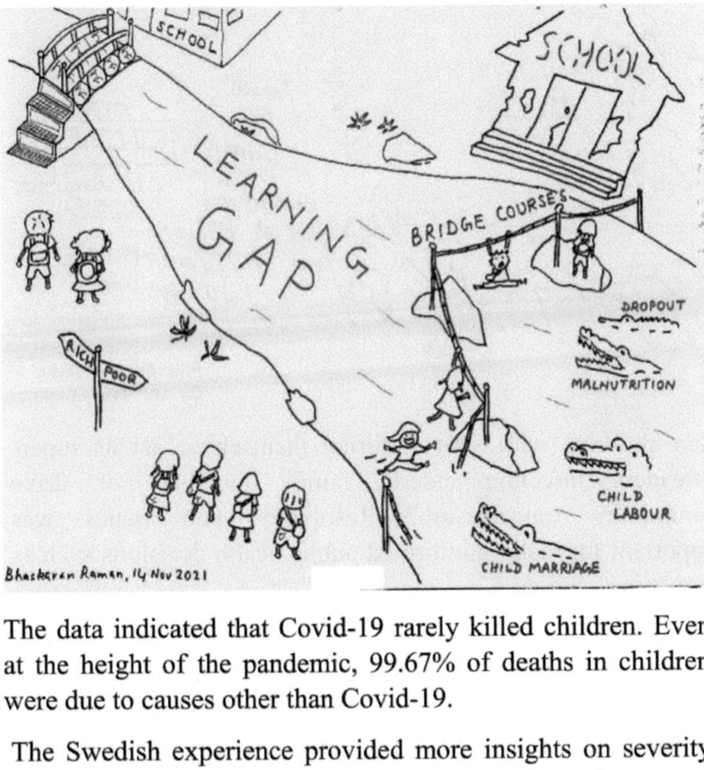

The data indicated that Covid-19 rarely killed children. Even at the height of the pandemic, 99.67% of deaths in children were due to causes other than Covid-19.

The Swedish experience provided more insights on severity of Covid-19 in children. Sweden was perhaps the only country to keep schools and preschools open during the course of the pandemic. A study by Karolinska Institute among Swedish schoolchildren who were seriously affected by Covid-19 has been published in the New England Journal of Medicine. They found that serious Covid-19, defined as needing treatment in an intensive care unit (ICU), was rare among school children despite schools being open during the pandemic. Only 1 child in 130,000 was treated in an ICU during the four month period of the study. A total of 15 children were admitted in the ICU. Seven of them had multi-inflammatory syndrome (MIS-C), which has been linked to Covid-19. Four of them had underlying disease. None of the children died. The most common time in the ICU was 4 days.

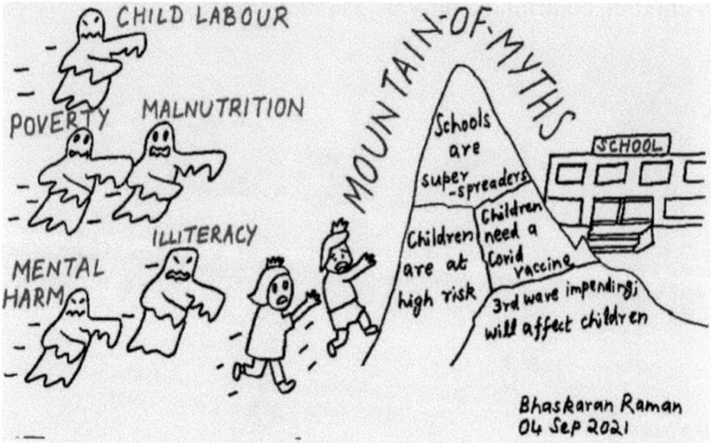

Can children, while not suffering themselves, act as super-spreaders infecting elderly family members or drive community transmission? Resolving such issues was important for making informed public health decisions such as reopening schools.

An overview of the available evidence in the peer reviewed journal, Pediatrics, titled, "“Covid-19 Transmission and Children: The Child Is Not to Blame,”" was reassuring. Studies of dynamics of Covid-19 transmission within families revealed that in majority of cases, the child developed symptoms after adults in the household, suggesting that the child was not the source of infection and that children most frequently acquired Covid-19 from adults rather than transmitting to them. Similar findings were reported from China.

What about transmission in schoolchildren spilling over to the community? The above overview on the basis of available evidence concludes that transmission in schools is less important in community transmission of Covid-19 than initially feared. This is in sharp contrast to influenza, for which transmission among schoolchildren is well established as a driver of community transmission.

The second wave which came like a bolt from the blue left us shaken and stirred. Apprehension of a third wave affecting children was understandable against this background. This delayed reopening of schools and colleges. All available evidence suggested that we could have moved cautiously forward and give a serious thought to reopening schools to avoid long term educational, social and psychological setbacks among the young generation.

The Art of War against the wily coronavirus.

We should use vaccines judiciously. What works in a small, sparsely populated and developed country may not work in a large, densely populated and developing country. It may not be cost effective either.

Viral infections have been with us since long. Doctors since decades were reconciled to having no effective remedies against viral infections. Patient management revolved around symptomatic treatment. However, after the discovery of antibiotics many lives were saved which otherwise would have succumbed to secondary bacterial infections. Parallels are drawn, generating panic, between the present pandemic and the influenza pandemic of 1918. The flu pandemic in 1918-1919 caused 50 million deaths at a time when the world population was 1.8 billion as against 7.8 billion currently. These figures are enough to cause mass hysteria.

However, this comparison is highly inappropriate for many reasons. The flu pandemic of 1918-19 occurred when no antibiotics were available to treat secondary bacterial infections a common complication of any viral pneumonia. Over the past century many scientific papers have confirmed this.

This was also a period of great hardships and deprivation in the aftermath of the First World War. It is not a coincidence that this pandemic of all times unfolded in the post war period. The global impact of the Great War on the overall health of people, along with lack of antibiotics, provided the ideal setting for devastations and deaths associated with it.

Over the next decades, medical advances, particularly the discovery of penicillin and other antibiotics which became freely available after the second war saved many lives, not only from bacterial diseases, but also from secondary infections following viral infections.

However, for decades, lethal viral diseases even in absence of secondary bacterial infections, continued to cause havoc. Smallpox epitomizes the agony and ecstasy of the human experience with viral infections. It had a case fatality rate of 30% and 80% of the survivors had deep pitted scars, or pockmarks. Some went blind. This was the agony of smallpox. Comparing smallpox with the novel coronavirus would be like comparing Hitler with Gandhi.

The moment of ecstasy for public health was the eradication of smallpox in 1980. However, the history of this victory spans centuries, not decades or years. It all started in 1796 when Edward Jenner, an astute observer, noted that milkmaids who recovered from cowpox never contacted smallpox. To test this hypothesis, he inoculated material from cowpox sore into the arm of a nine year boy James Phipps. Subsequently, Jenner exposed the boy to smallpox virus but the child never contacted the disease. No present day institutional review board would give an ethical approval to such a study!

From the discovery of the smallpox vaccine to eradication, the journey was exceedingly slow, as if travelling by horse cart (called Tonga in Hindi), of an earlier era. It took more than 200 years and a worldwide vaccination program to eradicate it. Smallpox was the first and to this day remains the last disease of global public health importance to be eradicated.

Besides having a really effective vaccine (no masks or physical distancing were needed after vaccination), there were a number of factors which enabled the eradication of this human scourge.

No sophisticated tests were needed to detect smallpox; even a lay person could identify it. There were no asymptomatic cases or hidden carriers who could transmit to others unknowingly. The virus was confined to humans and never infected animals or survived in the environment for long.

In spite of it being highly lethal, the smallpox virus was straightforward lacking the guile of most viruses such as the poliovirus or the SARS-CoV-2 which generate a large number of hidden infections. Straightforwardness takes neither humans nor viruses far. This enabled the eradication of the smallpox virus.

On the other hand, the novel coronavirus, having its origins in China, is true to the teachings of Sun Tzu. This warrior-philosopher from China, wrote The Art of War, 2000 years ago. Sun Tzu emphasized the role of deception in war, 'A military operation involves deception. Even though you are competent, appear to be incompetent, though effective, appear to be ineffective...When you are going to attack nearby, make it look as if you are far away...' This deception was aptly illustrated by the unexpected second wave in India!

The world gave the virus a chase and rightly so. Had the efforts been successful, this virus would have been nipped in the bud. With each passing day, the virus got deeply entrenched in the community aided by all the deception at its command. We had to reconcile to a low intensity long drawn conflict.

From smallpox virus to the coronavirus, we have come a long way. Vaccines which took centuries, decades and years to be rolled out in the community have been developed within a year an unthinkable and laudable feat. Extraordinary advances in genomics and precision medicine have driven this miracle in vaccine production. In record time we thought we had a strong weapon against the SARS-CoV-2 virus.

To get a level playing field against this deceptive and strong enemy, we too should have taken lessons from Sun Tzu's Art of War which cautions about use of strong weapons with these words, "Therefore, those who are not thoroughly aware of the disadvantages in the use of arms cannot be thoroughly aware of the advantages in the use of arms."

Taking heed of this, we should have preserved our ammunition, the vaccine and used it judiciously. Like a good general, we should have surveyed the lay of the land. What works in a small, sparsely populated and developed country may not work in a large, densely populated and developing county. Moreover, it may not be cost effective either.

Evidence kept accumulating that natural infection was robust and comparable to vaccine induced immunity, if not better. Densely populated countries like India with congested slums and tenements, and congested marketplaces, where social distancing is difficult, provide ideal conditions for fast community transmission of natural infection, before the vaccine can reach them. The fast rise of the second wave is testimony to that.

The key to community control of viral infections is herd immunity. This can be obtained either by natural infections, slowly, or by vaccines, swiftly. Natural herd immunity can be compared to the tonga (horse-cart of a bygone era), while vaccine immunity can be compared to a modern motorized bus.

Data from some parts of the country indicated that large swathes of the population had developed antibodies against SARS-CoV2 in the aftermath of the second wave. In Ahmedabad in Gujarat, one of the worst affected states, more than 70% of the population were found positive for antibodies in the last week of May 2021, a sharp rise from the 28% detected in February 2021.

Recently, the nonagenarian thespian, Dilip Kumar was in the news. It reminded one of his movie Naya Daur made in 1957. The story is set in a village where the main mode of transport is the *tonga* or horse cart. The hero is a *tongawallah* (horse-cart rider). The livelihoods of the tongawallahs are threatened when entrepreneurs from the city come to introduce buses in the village. There is much dispute and it is decided that to resolve it there would be a race between the *tonga* and the bus.

Under normal conditions, the bus would have easily outrun the *tonga*. However, in the climax of the movie the *tonga* wins the race as it was more negotiable under village conditions.

Repeated serosurveys in pandemics have an important role. This is crucial not only for predicting future waves, but also to guide vaccination strategy. Based on the findings and the logistics of mass vaccination a more targeted vaccine policy may give the bang for the buck. Excluding people with antibodies and including only the susceptible would have achieved herd immunity faster at minimum cost. In highly dense countries like India, the *tonga* of naturally acquired herd immunity will tend to be ahead of the bus carrying vaccines.

The Science and Art of Living with Covid

Science to deal with Covid had been brilliant but the Art was missing. We should have followed the strategy of Chess, which combines both science and art of looking at big picture to decide when a draw is better

'"Ars longa, vita brevis,"' is the translation into Latin of a part of quotation by the Greek '"Father of Medicine"' - Hippocrates. The English translation of this phrase is '"Art is long, life is short."' Fully translated from the Greek, the quote goes, '"Art is long, life is short, opportunity fleeting, experience perilous, and decision difficult. The pandemic drove home vividly this ancient wisdom.'

While the 19th and 20th centuries witnessed scientific advances at a leisurely pace, the 21st century is witnessing these advances at breakneck speed. Computing, precision medicine, genomics, and informatics, are propelling these.

These rapid and remarkable advances seem to have come at the cost of the art. Medicine which was one of the oldest arts is increasing becoming the newest science. The purity of this new science is approaching the point of sterility. Hard science is objective and easily understood, the potential often overestimated. Art is subjective and abstract, its subtlety difficult to understand and its potential often underestimated. It encompasses (but not restricted to) the social sciences, ethics, empathy and concern for human dignity both in life and death.

The pandemic from its genesis to its onward course, revealed brilliant science but deficient art. The finger of suspicion is pointed towards lab origin of the virus, an accident of '"gain of function"' research. '"Gain of function research"' aims to outpace nature ostensibly for research purposes. It is hazardous to say the least. The brilliance of science unleashed without the constraints of ethics and humanism has potential for immense harm like the misuse of nuclear power. Nuclear power went astray during the Second World War with devastating consequences. Was the pandemic the result of biological power gone astray? As the dust settles we may get the answers, hopefully.

The dilution of the art of medicine has also influenced epidemiology – the study of disease dynamics in population – a vital tool for control of pandemics. Earlier epidemiologists did field and house to house visits more than even postmen. This helped them to collect data first hand and also study the social and cultural factors (social epidemiology) in a population which are major determinants of disease dynamics. The art was known as '"shoe-leather epidemiology."' The classic example is John Snow's investigations of the London outbreak of cholera in 1854. Over the years, epidemiologists, particularly those in academics, became less enterprising and '"shoe-leather epidemiology"' gave way to '"arm-chair epidemiology."' Social epidemiology took a back seat.

Presently we are in the era of big data. Data mining and mathematical models contribute to understanding of many epidemiological issues. However, it has spawned a generation of '"mouse-click epidemiologists"' completely ignorant of social epidemiology. The harsh measures in response to the present pandemic based on sterile mathematical models, illustrates the consequences of neglect of social epidemiology.

Mouse-click epidemiology predicted large number of deaths as well as generated evidence for drastic measures such as school closures and physical distancing extending to lockdowns. The latter was based on a computer project for influenza control by a high school student, strange, but true. Building on this school project, scientists in the US ran hypothetical data into supercomputers framing policies reminiscent of the Middle Ages! Strategies such as school closure, physical distancing and lockdowns based on these outputs were named '"non-pharmacological interventions (NPI)."'

Lacking insights in social epidemiology, human beings were taken as inert units in the model rather than social beings. Elegant computer outcomes indicated that such drastic measures would break the "chain of transmission."' Both the prediction and NPI models went wide off the mark as evidenced by much low fatalities worldwide then projected, and the virus travelling from China to Chandni Chowk.

The art of medicine since the times of Hippocrates cautioned '"First do no harm."' The cure should not be worse than the malady. Blind science neglected this axiom. The collateral damages due to the sterile science are immense. Loss of livelihoods leads to severe malnutrition, increase in infectious diseases and deaths from other causes. The harm exceeded the benefit of lives saved from Covid-19. In the blind chase for the coronavirus we have sacrificed a lot, human dignity as well as human life.

The latest scientific miracle has been the development of vaccines against Covid-19 in record time. The euphoria of this has raised the hope of immediate eradication.

In chess, the '"hardest thing to win is a won game."' This was stated by an artist of the game, Emmanuel Lasker, a mathematician, philosopher and World Chess Champion for 27 years. An ambitious goal of eradicating Covid-19, which the world medical community appears to have ventured upon, is as tough as winning a won game. We have the winning piece, the vaccine in record time, a laudable feat. However, as in chess, more important than the winning pieces are the right moves.

The pandemic played out across the globe in varying patterns. Every game of chess has the same pieces but different combination of moves depending on the situation in each game. Thanks to brilliant science, we have a robust surveillance and monitoring system, and treatment protocols have been refined. All these with the vaccine, make for heavy arsenal against the virus. The efforts of researchers, laboratory scientists, and clinicians assembling these pieces are commendable.

If we miss the art at this juncture, we will lose the game. While the science will tend to advocate mass vaccination, the art should see the big picture. Should we go for a win or a draw? History of medicine does not have any account of eradication of any disease in such short time. Like in chess, it is very difficult to win a won game. The efficacy of vaccines is also mired in uncertainty. Given these imponderables, it would be more pragmatic to opt for a draw and learn to live with Covid-19. Once we vaccinate the vulnerable of all ages, and the elderly, Covid-19 should cease to be a public health problem in India.

You are as healthy as you think you are.

Anxiety, panic and loss of livelihood was bound to trigger a wave of diseases other than Covid. Instead of taking harsh measures, policymakers needed to adapt to the stages of the pandemic as it evolved

The French philosopher Rene Descartes rejected the notion that mind and body are connected. Descartes dismissed the idea that mind influences physical health. He speculated that mind comprises unidentifiable and immaterial substance so it cannot affect the body which is solid matter. Gilbert Ryle nailed it further by labelling the non-physical mind as the "Ghost in the Machine."

Western medicine adopted the separation proposed by Descartes. It also found it easier to fix a mechanical body without having to deal with the enigmatic, "Ghost in the Machine."

Nevertheless, physicians down the ages are aware of the placebo effect contributing to the healing process. Placebo effect is when people get better when they believe (falsely) that they are getting an effective drug. Conversely there is a nocebo effect, i.e. negative thinking about an illness or therapy, can adversely affect health. So in practice, mind does affect the body.

Fiction writers free from constraints of scientific consensus often get it right. Two centuries after Descartes discarded the mind body connection, O Henry elegantly narrates the nocebo and placebo effects in his classic short story '"The Last Leaf."'

Set against the background of an epidemic of pneumonia, the story deals with mind body connection. Down with a nasty bout of pneumonia, the patient, a young lady, is full of negativity and impending doom of death. The view from her window is bare and dreary. She could see a brick house around which an old ivy vine climbed up, its leaves rapidly falling in the autumn. She keeps counting the remaining ones. This symbolises the ebbing of life from her body. The falling leaves act as nocebo. She passively waits for death believing it will coincide with the fall of the last leaf. Her doctor gives up hope. The penultimate day arrives. Only one leaf remains. There is strong wind and heavy rain throughout the night.

An aging neighbour, a failed artist comes to know about her. He paints a leaf on the wall across. It turns out to be the only masterpiece he has ever painted. Next day the lady sees the sole leaf standing in spite of the heavy winds and rain throughout the night. This gives her the will to fight and live. The painted leaf acts as a placebo. She recovers. The aging artist exposed to the elements succumbs to pneumonia.

While O Henry in his short story may have conveyed the mind body as a work of fiction there is emerging evidence albeit nebulous of mind body connection. Fiction and fact seem to be merging.

The concept of salutogenesis by Antonovsky, in the twentieth century, described in his book Health, Stress and Coping, suggests that life experiences help shape one's sense of coherence making it comprehensible, meaningful and manageable. This helps one to cope with stress. More recently, Martin Seligman distinguished between flourishing and languishing persons. Flourishing persons experience more positive feelings, while languishing persons have more negative ones.

These phenomena not only shape mental well being, but also have impact on physical health both short term and long term. In the short term stressors reduce immunity to infections, while in the long run they may be risk factors for heart diseases, high blood pressure, diabetes, other endocrine disorders, autoimmune disorders, skin disorders and psychiatric illnesses.

It is a well known experience among students that acute stress of examinations increases bouts of common cold suggesting some inhibition of natural immunity. Research also suggests that psychological stressors increase risk of acute infectious respiratory illnesses.

Studies in the field of psycho-neuro-immunology, which explores the interactions between stressors and immunity through release of chemical hormones, are still evolving. They encounter difficulties as both stress and immunity are multifaceted and difficult to measure.

Easier to understand is how stressors may impact immunity and health in indirect ways. Stress as a result of prolonged panic from pandemics drive people to unhealthy food, tobacco and alcohol (witness the long queues at liquor shops during relaxation of lockdowns). All these while lowering immunity in the short term increas the risk of chronic diseases. People losing their livelihoods suffer from malnutrition reducing the immunity to infections.

Whether direct or indirect the effect of panic induced stress in the pandemic was highly detrimental to public health. The effects may be seen in the long run with higher rate of mental illness, alcoholism, substance abuse, chronic diseases while in the short run large number of people will be susceptible to infectious diseases due to low immunity.

The common strategy of most governments in the pandemic was to instil fear in people. This strategy was been used in a paternalistic manner to make people compliant to "covid appropriate behaviour." This approach may have been justified in the initial uncertain stages of the pandemic as a precautionary principle to err on the side of safety. This resulted in prolonged panic of populations and mass hysteria. Short term stress transformed into long term stress for many. Mostly these measures were inappropriate and the chronic stress due to suspended businesses, education, recreation and associated uncertainties caused immense harm due to adverse impact on mental, physical and social wellbeing of people. While mathematical modellers continued to predict future waves, , it does not require rocket science to predict a colossal wave of chronic mental and other non-covid diseases against a background of severe malnutrition as a result of extreme measure to control an uncontrollable virus which has an infection fatality rate of around 0.1% in our country.

As in the Bhagwad-Gita, we should have adapted to the stages of the pandemic as it evolved. First there was “‘“tamas”’” (darkness, destruction and chaos) when nothing was know about the novel coronavirus and many fatalities were due to chaotic mismanagement; then there was “‘“rajas”’” (passion, action, confusion), the passion of scientists to fight the virus at all costs, actions which were sometimes inappropriate and confusing messages from experts; while subsequently we should have moved on to “‘“sattva”’” (goodness, constructive action, harmony) and learned to live with the virus. This is the way forward to rescue the world from the global panic and mass obsessive compulsive disorder.

Diverting resources and time to Covid to the exclusion of other health issues poor policy.

A nation does not become healthy by vaccines alone. We need a much better public health system, safe drinking water, nutrition and much else. Diverting most resources to Covid-19 was just not good policy

India is a fast developing economy. It has a burgeoning middle class with rising aspirations. It is moving towards capitalism and free market economy. Freed from the shackles of socialism, the economy is speeding like a fast car. However, if the roads are poorly maintained with unreliable traffic signals, fast cars can cause accidents, occasionally running over people on pavements.

In the last seven decades, the number of vehicles on Indian roads has risen by 11% every year. The road network on the other hand has grown by only 4% yearly – a gross mismatch. While responsible for traffic jams, increasing private transport on Indian roads has benefitted neither the rich nor the poor. Both suffer from increasing air pollution, traffic snarls and road traffic accidents, which kill over 400 people every day in India and maim over 1200 more, mostly young people.

The risk of a young person dying from road traffic accident in India is many times more than the probability of dying from Covid-19. If these counts are projected every day with gory images of accident victims by 24 x 7 news channels and social media, one can imagine the panic it will cause.

A permanent solution to traffic problems can only be achieved by increasing the quality of public transport in the country which is in a pathetic state. Gustavo Petro, the former Mayor of Bogota had remarked, "“A developed country is not a place where the poor have cars. It is where the rich use public transportation.”"

The expanding middle class while pursuing their dreams for a better life tend to neglect their health. Most have little time for physical activity and home cooked healthy foods. Increased sedentariness and fast foods lead to lifestyle conditions like diabetes, hypertension, coronary heart disease and obesity. The current pandemic illustrates that these lifestyle diseases also make people more vulnerable to Covid-19.

Living in the fast lane increases the demand not only for new cars but also a pill for every ill and newer vaccines even if they are on trial mode like new cars with temporary registration numbers.

Newer vaccines can definitely prevent diseases and deaths from a number of conditions depending on local epidemiology and public health problems. Vaccines in poor countries have had extraordinary successes as well as severe setbacks. There is a fundamental difference between vaccines which are administered to healthy people and drugs which are given to diseased patients. Adverse effects due to vaccines in healthy however rare, raises concerns of safety, ethics and public trust. Overlooking these aspects can erode trust leading to vaccine hesitancy. This can adversely impact vaccination programs.

Just as good roads and monitoring of traffic rules are essential to prevent road traffic accidents, good monitoring and surveillance systems should be in place to prevent vaccine related accidents and adverse events from an ever increasing number of newer vaccines developed and introduced at warp speed.

With our existing limitations of public health infrastructure this will be difficult. Fast tracking mass vaccination without proper infrastructure can be hazardous. It would be like running a superfast train on old rickety tracks.

Most vulnerable will be the marginalized and poor people in rural and remote regions out of range of a surveillance system for reporting adverse events following immunization. Their vulnerability can be compared to pavement dwellers who are at risk of being run over by fast cars.

Introduction of a new vaccine like the Covid-19, can also impact the routine childhood immunization program and can overstretch the creaking public health system. Scant resources are likely to be diverted from care of other neglected diseases in our country which have higher morbidity and mortality. Every day about 25,000 people die in India from various causes. Tuberculosis takes a daily toll of 1200 persons in spite of having a vaccine for it which too claims to reduce severity and deaths; 2000 children die every day in our country from preventable diseases; typhoid is endemic in spite of an effective vaccine and treatment, to name a few.

Compared to burden of other communicable diseases in our country, Covid-19 with an infection fatality rate between 0.1 to 0.3% pales into insignificance, as between 99.9 to 99.7% of people infected with the novel corona virus survive. Our endemic diseases with higher morbidity and mortality hardly get a fraction of the resources for their surveillance and control compared to Covid-19. Our priorities should be decided by our public health problems instead of Western models.

The latest round of serosurvey in our country revealed that 67% or 90 crores Indians have already encountered the novel coronavirus. Studies from all over show that people who have recovered from natural infection have long lasting and robust immunity even after waning of the antibody levels.

The government allocated Rs 35, 000 crores for 150 crores doses of Covid-19 vaccine which can vaccinate 75 crores. Going by the science and current evidence regarding the effectiveness and duration of natural immunity we could have opted out of mass vaccination to avoid duplicating this population level immunity conferred by nature. It was like giving a breast fed baby top milk.

Instead, we could have resorted to smart vaccination by focused protection of people with comorbidities and elderly. This way we could have saved a huge amount from the Rs 35,000 crores allotted for the mass vaccination campaign diverting this for other pressing public health problems. For instance water and sanitation was allotted just Rs 21, 158 crores. A large burden of disease in our country is related to water and sanitation.

We can sum up by saying that a good health will be achieved not only by vaccines. It will be achieved by good public health infrastructure, safe water, nutrition, housing, and clean environment and judicious use of vaccines.

No difference between medicine and T20 cricket.

Like cricket, the practice of medicine has now been commercialized, glamorized and turned into spectator sport

In a bygone era, Test matches were the most popular form of cricket. Those were the days of the transistor, not television. School and college students, office workers and executives, had their ears glued to pocket transistors for ball by ball commentary spanning over 5 days. The players wore whites, gentlemanly in attire and attitude. Few played for money or to become rich. They never signed contracts for commercials. There were no rich sponsors. Cricket was as pure as the whites worn by the players, without any "'conflicts of interest.'" The umpires' decision, even if wrong was taken as final sportingly. There were no third umpires.

Enter Kerry Packer, the Australia media mogul in the late seventies. Being first and foremost a money man, he lured the players with lucre and fame paving the way for one day internationals (ODIs) replacing test. The abandonment of whites by the players symbolized loss of innocence. From a gentleman's game, cricket got transformed into a spectator sport. Next to come was T20 cricket, the most popular form. The complexities and nuances of test cricket, appealing to the purist, seemed a legacy of a bygone era with dwindling fan following. High stakes driven by commercial interests, brought in third umpires and action replays.

Decades ago, the family physician or the general practitioner was sufficient for a lifetime of medical care. His/her accumulated knowledge and skills were acquired by first hand clinical experience of seeing real world patients in real world settings. He/she had an ear to the ground and could customise treatment according to the patient's background. Diagnosis was made by history taking and clinical examination with minimum of tests. The wisdom, intuition and skills these physicians acquired were beyond what could be learned between the covers of a textbook. And like the test cricketers of yesteryears these good doctors earned more fame than fortune. The doctor knew best. There were few litigations or incidences of violence against doctors.

Over the last few decades, the landscape of medical practice like that of cricket has changed. Advances in technology have made medical care costly, both for individuals and the state. It has brought about "'dislocations wrought by science,"' with emphasis on specialization. The pride of place of the family physician got usurped by the specialists and super-specialists, some acquiring the status of "'celebrity doctors."' Patient got impatient (pun intended), with high expectations of quick relief. Craving for instant results both in cricket and in medicine, has become a sign of quixotic times.

With advances in medical technology, the doctor-patient relationship diluted. Machines are replacing humans. Corporatization of medical services has given rise to a rapidly growing industry phasing out private clinics. Most doctors have to work in corporate hospitals surrendering autonomy. From a noble profession and a calling, medicine has become a big business.

Multiple stakeholders generate multiple conflicts of interest. As with present day cricket, commerce is influencing modern medical practice and policy. Even academic research has not been spared. High profile journals like the Lancet had to retract a highly publicized paper on Covid-19 which was based on fake data, reminiscent of "'match-fixing"' allegations against some famous cricketers.

The pandemic of Covid-19 laid bare the fault-lines which have developed due to commercialization of medicine; in practice, research and policy. The massive second wave of Covid-19 in India demonstrated the limitations of the corporate model of health care in dealing with emergencies. Lacking a good public health infrastructure, meagre hospital facilities were overwhelmed by numbers and not by the lethality of the virus.

Given the non-existent health facilities in rural areas, Covid-19 patients had to travel to over-stretched urban hospitals aggravating the chaos.

Commercial interests and politics influenced research and policy as well according to an editorial in the prestigious British Medical Journal. Career scientists and academics were influenced by conflicts of interest. Policies for Covid-19 control were finalized on advice of "‘celebrity clinicians’" instead of public health specialists and epidemiologists. Medicine became a spectator sport like T20 cricket. Vaccines which used to take decades for development got ready within a year, a laudable feat. When earlier vaccines were administered on advice of the family physician, during the pandemic they were being promoted by celebrity film stars and cricketers to eliminate "‘vaccine hesitancy.’" This is reminiscent of promotion of cola drinks by celebrity cricketers and film stars, an innovative and efficient adaptation of social marketing, laudable.

Diseases do not read textbooks. In every disease, there are outlier cases which fascinate the clinicians and discussed at length at professional conferences and published in reputed journals. Over the years, the perception of clinicians is distorted by these outliers which become the norm for them. Present day media joins in highlighting such outliers which attract attention. This highlighting distorts the public perception too who continue to be in perpetual panic mode due to these serious but rare outcomes of a normally self limiting disease. Public health policy should be dictated by the less fascinating majority of cases, the normal distribution, so to say. However, this neither draws attention nor brings fame. The fact is that the novel coronavirus in India has an infection fatality rate of 0.1% or less. One has to do trade-offs in balancing scarce resources around this figure. This is sound public health practice albeit taking away the glamour of a quixotic battle against a novel virus.

A famous physician hailing from a family of doctors in ancient China was once asked who among his brothers is the most famous. He answered, "'My eldest brother sees the spirit of sickness and removes it before it takes shape, so his name does not go out of the house; my second brother cures the sickness in its very early stages, so his name does not go out of the neighbourhood; as for me, I puncture veins, prescribe potions, and massage skin, and so from time to time my name gets out and is heard among the lords.'"

Someone from a bygone era may say – This is not Cricket!

It's time to think 'slow' now.

Governments took the pandemic for a sprint event, where unthinking speed was the essence. It is turning out to be a marathon which demands stamina, endurance and planning

Nobel Laureate Daniel Kahneman coined the phrase, "'thinking fast and slow.'" Thinking fast is intuitive and effortless, while thinking slow is deliberate and calls for effort. After "'thinking fast,'" taking time out for "'thinking slow'" can be worthwhile.

The response to the pandemic was driven by panic. Fear of imminent danger led to thinking fast. Governments were like students attempting questions out of their syllabus. In the manner of unprepared students, they resorted to mass copying. Country after country copied Communist China's draconian measures, the imitators outdoing the trendsetter.

Fast thinking led to contradictions, as they usually do. Initially there were conflicting messages regarding use of face mask by the general public. The WHO also made a U-turn after announcing that asymptomatic persons do not transmit the virus. And then there was backtracking by the WHO after announcing that asymptomatic people need not be tested. None of these statements are right or wrong but need to be considered in proper context. Pandemic evolves in stages. What is applicable in one region at any time may not be applicable in another region which may be in a different stage of the pandemic.

Responding to disease outbreaks is a dynamic process like driving a car. Taking off from a stationary position one has to engage the fuel intensive first gear. Once on the run, fuel is preserved by engaging top gears. At the end of the drive, once again, fuel intensive lower gears are used. Outbreak response also follows a similar sequence. Intensive containment measures should be applied when the outbreak starts to take off, once the outbreak breaks into community transmission, intensive containment measures are not very cost-effective. The strategy at this stage should change gears to control fatalities by ensuring early management of cases leaving the asymptomatic well alone. When the disease is on verge of eradication, again containment measures such as test, trace and isolation become important and would include testing of asymptomatic contacts as well.

Strangely it appears that except for the effortless panic driven "'fast thinking"' responses by most countries, what was lacking was deliberate "'slow thinking"' to consider the stage of the pandemic in a particular region to enable calibration of the response. We kept driving in the fuel intensive first gear.

The sprint is long over. It is time to abandon "'fast thinking."' Currently we are running a marathon. It is time for second wind and some "'thinking slow."' Having lost the sprint, we should endeavour to win the marathon. To be successful, we should let go of the measures which were appropriate for the sprint and adopt measures appropriate for a marathon.

Being well into community transmission, containment measures such as intensive testing and tracing particularly of asymptomatics should be discontinued. It makes no sense for requiring RT-PCR tests for inter-state travel either.

This will go a long way in allaying the fear and stigma of the disease. Another important step should be proper "'risk communication"' to the people. The modus operandi of most governments has been to instil fear in people to make them compliant to so called "'covid appropriate behaviour."' Without proper risk communication, most "'covid appropriate behaviour"' driven by "'fast thinking"' has degenerated into rituals with little impact on disease transmission. Superstars preaching and practicing these covid appropriate behaviours have contacted the virus themselves! This should make us take a pause and appraise the evidence base for these measures.

One example of covid ritualism is the advice not to step out of the house and wearing of masks if going outdoors. The origin of this guideline, as reported in New York Times, dated May 26, 2021, is interesting. The Centre for Disease Control (CDC), US, misinterpreted a scientific paper to conclude that the risk of outdoor transmission is 10%. In response to this misguided guideline, the corresponding author of this paper tweeted that the actual risk of outdoor transmission is 0.1%. In fact, in her tweet she recommended to spend more time outdoors to stay healthy mentioning that risk of outdoor transmission is negligible.

This misunderstanding led to restriction of outdoor activities worldwide. Many people who conduct businesses outdoors, such as vendors, street food and terrace restaurant owners could have continued to earn their livelihoods with minimal risk of transmission.

Risk communication should consider covid-19 in context. Globally, the risk of dying from infection with the virus is 0.3%, in India it is 0.1%. If someone in our country catches the virus, the probability of surviving is 99.9%. Living exposes us to much higher risks: daily 1500 Indians die from tuberculosis, 400 young people die every day from road traffic accidents (and 10 times more maimed for life), and 2000 children die daily from preventable diseases to give a few examples.

The majority of covid-19 infections are asymptomatic. Interim results released in June 2021, from a joint AIIMS-WHO study, indicates that 60-70% of the population, including children, have encountered the novel virus. Other studies in some parts of the country have revealed IgG antibodies in 80% of the population. Studies worldwide indicate that natural infection give robust and long lasting immunity. After infection, the virus replicates and circulates in our body for 10-15 days giving enough chance to familiarize our immune system including long acting memory and T cells. This immune memory logically should work against variants too. We recognize people whom we had known for some time, even after gap of many years from some residual features in their appearance.

The evidence and logic of not duplicating nature's efforts of natural immunity could have enabled population level immunity faster with minimum inputs, by using a "'smart vaccination"' strategy. If we had excluded people with IgG antibodies, we may have had to vaccinate only a fraction of our population saving lot of resources and money.

Our policy makers need to do some serious "'thinking slow,"' keeping politics and conflicts of interests at bay. Asking too much?

War Against Covid: No real winners here.

Draconian measures caused death in the developing world to prolong lives in the developed world

To prevent a bigger disaster than Covid-19, the world should have called off its "'Till We Win"' War against the novel coronavirus. Ashoka felt remorse and intense personal anguish after winning the Kalinga War, when he saw the deaths and devastations in the aftermath of the war.

Similarly, the Chinese warrior-philosopher Sun Tzu advised, "'He who wishes to fight must first count the cost. When you engage in actual fighting, if victory is long in coming, the men's weapons will grow dull and their ardour will be dampened. If you lay siege to a town, you will exhaust your strength."' He goes on to say, "'In the wise leader's plans, consideration of advantage and disadvantage will be blended together. "'

In Mahabharata, the victory in war for the Pandavas turned to desolation and despair when they witnessed the field of glory turn into a field of the dead and dying.

In declaring a war on Covid-19, the world bit off more than it could chew. Hasty decisions taken under panic did not weigh the death and desolation from collateral harm. The worst affected were people in low income countries. Heavy handed covid-19 control measures are not egalitarian. According to a paper in Lancet by Broadbent and colleagues, the costs fall on the global poor. Draconian measures cause deaths in the developing world to prolong lives in the developed world the authors concluded. This "'social distance"' between rich and poor is far greater than the "'physical distance"' needed for "'covid appropriate behaviour."' This "'social distance"' can decide life or death for the poor.

The war against Covid-19 had devastating impact on livelihoods, which threatened to jeopardize overall health of the majority of world citizens. The negative impact on public health will be far more than any modest impact towards control of the novel coronavirus. Endemic diseases particularly in low income tropical countries will flare up as most health resources were diverted towards control of Covid-19 on war footing.

India went for the largest and most complete lockdown in the world. An estimated 10 million migrant workers returned to their villages, many on foot, and some on bicycles. Poverty, unemployment and destitution were the fallout of such a drastic and hasty strategy. No fancy mathematical models were required to predict that we were facing a devastating social and economic disruption. An estimated 400 million people are at of risk falling into poverty.

In the 1962 war against China, our military inadequacies were exposed. In the current war against the China originated novel coronavirus, inadequacies in our public health infrastructure were laid bare. Care of non-covid cases, which cause many time more deaths from Covid-19, suffered. This was due to overwhelmed health services and reduced utilization. Even patients with serious non-covid conditions feared to visit hospital out of fear of catching covid. Recent estimates put a far higher number of excess deaths in India during the pandemic implying that the deaths from Covid-19 are being underreported. However, given the prevailing "'war-like"' environment with curfews more stringent than even during wartime, a large proportion of these excess deaths could have been due to non-covid conditions. During war there is "'noise"' and "'heat and dust"' along with propaganda obfuscating the true facts and figures. Dissent is not entertained or censored to win the war. Similar war-like strategies were used by world governments in this pandemic.

Medical, paramedical and frontline workers turned into corona-warriors. Being the foot soldiers in this war, they bore the brunt. While cheered with banging of thalis and lighting of diyas, often they faced stigma in society out of fear of contagion. This had a toll on their mental health and many suffered burnout. Some contacted and succumbed to the infection being exposed to high viral load in overcrowded hospitals.

Most things went on war-footing except for one curious exception. Medical students were sent home, medical teaching went online distancing the medical students from real world patients. While doctors, some elderly, went about their "'essential duties"', medical schools were closed ostensibly to shelter the young medical students who are much less vulnerable to the virus. This was a paradox. Imagine shutting down the National Defence Academy (NDA) or the Indian Military Academy (IMA) during a war!

Besides medical education which was suspended weakening the foundation of future health care, other educational institutions were shut down for more than two years. This will cause long term social, psychological and educational setback in the next generation.

Did all these drastic measures work? The available data do not provide evidence of success of these extraordinary measures implemented on a war footing. After the first wave of the pandemic in India, the country wide seropositivity according to Indian Council of Medical Research (ICMR) survey was 21%. After the second wave, the latest round of serosurvey by the ICMR reveal that about 67% or more than 90 crores of Indians had encountered the novel coronavirus (this should make it novel no more). The only silver lining is that this monumental denominator dilutes the Infection Fatality Rate to less than 0.1% in India. If someone contracts the virus, the chances of survival is about 99.9%. The infection fatality rate according to the Centre for Disease Control, USA is around 0.3%. So even if we correct for gross underreporting in India as is being alleged, the fatality from Covid-19 is much lower than most endemic communicable as well as non-communicable diseases in our country.

At the end of the day, one may ask,. Was the all out war against Covid-19 worth the collateral harm? Or a low-intensity-conflict would have been desirable? Let us hope that sanity prevails and this all- out war "'Till We Win"' against Covid-19 is modified to a "'low-intensity-conflict"' commensurate to the lethality of the virus vis-a-vis our other pressing public health problems.

Panic and the Pandemic – Breaking free towards freedom of the mind

Independence day thoughts on science and art of spreading panic.

Where the mind is without fear and the head is held high;
Where knowledge is free;
Where the world has not been broken up into fragments
By narrow domestic walls;
Where words come out from the depths of truth;
Where tireless striving stretches its arms towards perfection;
Where the clear stream of reason has not lost its way;
Into the dreary dead sand of dead habit;
Where the mind is led forward by thee;
Into ever-widening thought and action;
Into that heaven of freedom,
My Father, let my country awake.
[Rabindranath Tagore]

As we celebrate the 75th Independence Day, the majority of our people are living in panic of the pandemic. In the current pandemic, the response of most world governments has added to the woes of the people. The world is facing a global ""'iatrogenic'"" disaster. The freedom and autonomy of people are also severely curtailed with every wave or the apprehension of a wave ostensibly for saving the people from the novel coronavirus. Frequent lockdowns are destroying livelihoods and in the long run, more people will die from poverty associated conditions than will be saved from Covid-19.

In this environment, the mind is full of fear and it is difficult to hold the head high.

What about knowledge? Knowledge, particularly scientific knowledge, thrives when opposite points of views and alternative hypotheses are debated and discussed. Great disagreements generate great science. History of medicine has many examples of doctors who did not conform to group-think and were ridiculed and dismissed as mavericks only later to be proved right.

Ignaz Semmelweiss, the Hungarian physician, in the nineteenth century based on meticulously collected data, advocated hand-washing to prevent infections which was responsible for high mortality after birth. In his lifetime, he was ridiculed and ostracised by the medical community who declared his inference, in spite of evidence, outlandish. Dejected, he took to alcohol and ended in an asylum in 1865 where he was beaten to death. He paid a heavy price for his courage of conviction. After more than a century and a half, the world is following his advice with gusto!

Professionals form powerful associations, which promote the status quo at times under the garb of "'medical consensus.'" Going against group-think is not easy and can endanger one's academic and scientific career. History is repeating itself. Any viewpoint against the present medical consensus is censored instead of being debated. Dogma is replacing debate. Science decays in such an environment.

In the era of "'grants driven research'", often the scientific script is influenced by the sponsors. Knowledge is not free. To acquire it through research, one needs research grants.

How to realize Tagore's dream of knowledge being free when research is possible only by grants from sponsors with vested interests? Perhaps one way can be more investment by the state in research. A corpus for research generated by unlinked anonymous donors from corporate business houses can also be considered.

The pandemic has broken up the world into fragments. The response to it led to severe travel restrictions. After the availability of vaccines, "'vaccine passports'" are being contemplated. Scientists questioning the safety and efficacy of vaccines are labelled as "'anti-vaxxers'" instead of rebutting them with evidence and hard data. This debate with evidence and hard data will also convince the people better and will remove "'vaccine hesitancy'" rather than propaganda and caller tunes. Alas, this clear stream of reason, envisaged by Tagore, has lost its way.

What is the way forward to clear the stream of reason and steer it towards the proper course?

Fear is generated by ignorance. Fuelled by media and vested interests the panic spreads like a forest fire faster than any virus. Population panic makes people vulnerable to exploitation by vested interests. Vested interests like the mass hysteria to be as prolonged as possible.

Regrettably, most countries, except for few notable examples like Sweden, treated people in a paternalistic manner rather than as free citizens. Like parents disciplining their child who invoke fear to make them behave in a desirable manner, governments, media and even academics, spread panic and fear, to coerce people to comply.

The vaccine for mass panic is risk communication. This should be transparent and informed. Creating panic and fear, with its offshoots of stigma and shaming and ridiculing is manipulation and not risk communication.

While scientists are exploring precision medicine to develop fast track vaccines, trace variants and their behaviour, a similar precision approach to risk communication is desirable to inform the people and eliminate panic.

People should be made to realise that daily we live with some amount of risk to life. This risk can never be reduced to zero. So if we wait for zero cases of covid we would be in perpetual lockdown and most of us will die of starvation before the virus reaches us. Similarly, like all respiratory viruses there will be seasonal fluctuations. These molehills can be converted into mountains by various forms of conflicts of interest.

Risk estimation which relies on science and judgment need to be emphasized for public information. Science of statistics can compile deaths in past waves to predict future calamities. Judgement involves social and political issues. It involves point of views of individuals and communities who face the risk. A trade off is always involved between perceived benefits and harms – this seems to have been overlooked by most world governments in this pandemic. The risk of dying after catching the coronavirus is 0.3% globally and lower in India because of younger population. Based on this hard data, it can be communicated to people that if a healthy person gets infected with the novel virus, chances of survival for that person is 99.7%. This survival is far higher than most of our endemic diseases. Even this risk is not uniform across the age strata. Healthy children have almost zero risk of dying from Covid-19.

Risk communication should also stress on the high risk groups such as people with co-morbidities, the frail elderly, and perhaps even younger people with co-morbidities. Focused protection can be advised for them while the healthy that face minimal risk can carry on their routine activities.

The implications of the results of the latest serosurvey by ICMR in which almost 67% of the population have shown to have protective IgG antibodies if properly communicated can also allay the population panic.

Let us hope that this Independence Day, reason and rationality leads us back "'into ever-widening thought and action; and into that heaven of freedom...'" envisaged by Tagore.

Healthwise: cost of chasing the impossible.

Panic and fear contributed to deaths due to COVID, confirm peer-reviewed research. Panic and wrong policies also allowed vested interests to push dubious cures and claim 99% efficacy!

"'Thor, the god of thunder and lightning, in Norse mythology, stood in front of the giant king. Pride was at stake. The king asked a drinking horn to be placed before Thor, challenging him to empty it. Thor picked up the goblet and took one long gulp after another but no matter how deeply and how much he drank, he found his breath running out with the drinking horn still almost full. He kept on making fast and furious attempts to drain the goblet but all in vain, the level did sink in the vessel but he could not empty it.'"

Thor was perplexed. Wrapped up in his own confusion, he did not notice the anxiety in the King's demeanour. What had been handed to Thor was not a simple goblet. By trickery, the horn was connected to the nearby ocean. And Thor had come close to draining the ocean! Unknowingly, he was attempting the impossible.

This story is from ancient mythology. Are we, in trying to drain the novel coronavirus from the globe, living a similar challenge as Thor faced while trying to drain the goblet? Are we too attempting the impossible?

Our country is an ocean of people and most have recovered from natural infection with the coronavirus. The recommended strategy of test, trace and isolate hardly made any dent on the spread of infection or identifying all with the infection. Only a fraction of infections were identified by these methods to "'break the chain of transmission'" and drain the reservoir of the virus in the community.

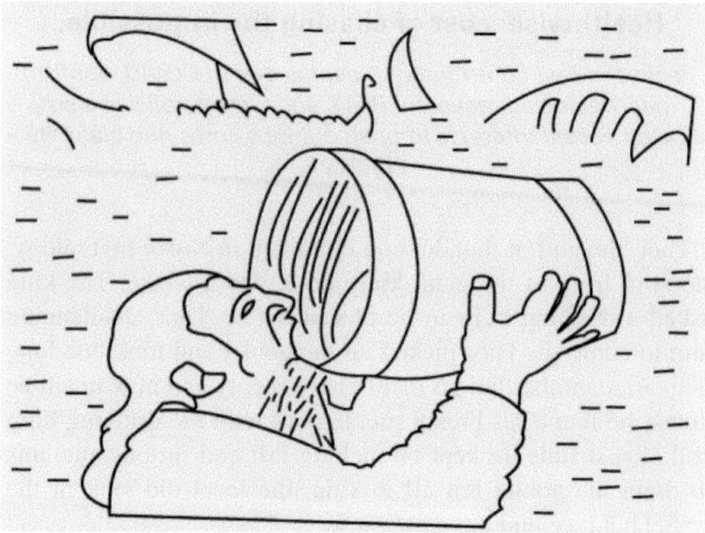

The June 2021 round of serosurvey conducted by Indian Council of Medical Research (ICMR), showed that 67.6% of Indians had antibodies. From this we can infer that a staggering 92 crores plus had developed immunity either due to natural infection, mostly, or partly due to vaccination. Around the time of the survey, less than 20% of the population had taken a single dose and around 5% had taken both doses of the vaccine. So we can assume that around 75 crores people in our country had acquired immunity from having recovered from natural infection. The cases identified by the "'test, treat, isolate"' strategy stood at a miniscule of around 3 crores. So by intense contact tracing efforts of Herculean proportions (or Thorian proportions!) we had been able to detect only 4% of cases in the country at this point of time.

The novel coronavirus is the don of all viruses, not only difficult but impossible to catch up with. And like all successful dons, it ruled more by fear and panic, rather than lethality alone. The panic and fear also contributed to deaths from this virus, as brought out in a recent peer reviewed original research paper published in the July 2021 issue of Public Health Research, Practice and Policy by Kompaniyets and colleagues. Among 540, 667 adults hospitalized with Covid-19, the researchers tried to identify the risk factors for severe outcomes and deaths. To their surprise the investigators, found anxiety and fear-related disorders to be the second highest risk factor after obesity leading to death from Covid-19.

Scientists advising the government lost the plot early. Testing and tracing are important in the early stages of an outbreak when it is a localised stream and has not merged into the ocean (of humanity), or at the end of the pandemic when it has reduced to a puddle, i.e. if the public health problem associated with the disease still demands eradication. Else the puddle can be left alone. We have so many un-cleared and bigger puddles in our country such as tuberculosis which kill over 1200 every day, child deaths – over 2000 daily, typhoid which does not have a proper surveillance and counting system in place but the estimated burden is appreciable in spite of an effective vaccine, and so on.

Not only the futility of it. What about the costs of these futile measures when the stream had merged with the ocean of community transmission? What about the opportunity costs? What about the fear, stigma and harassment of quarantine among those randomly picked up in the goblet while the bulk of those harbouring the virus were in the ocean of humanity in our densely populated country?

First, let us consider the futility and utility of testing and tracing. From the scientific perspective testing and tracing does not make any sense once community transmission has set in. Even if the number of tests had been increased 10 times still we would have missed the bulk of positive cases which occurred in our country as revealed by the latest serosurvey.

On the other hand, aggressive testing and tracing and quarantining have great utility to increase the case counts and generate panic and fear among the people. People harbour so many viruses and bacteria in their throat, gut and skin some of which cause far more serious diseases than Covid-19. But never in history of medicine were people labelled as cases on basis of disease-causing pathogens isolated from them without any symptoms as was done for Covid-19. The ensuing panic of rising case counts is exploited by vested interest to promote dubious treatments and preventives all assured of over 99% success rates given the low Infection Fatality Ratc of 0.3% of the "'lethal'" virus.

What about the costs? It has been estimated that the costs of contact tracing in the USA was 3.6 billion dollars. India's population is three times that of the USA so the approximate costs of contact tracing and quarantining in our country would be about 14 billion dollars. Can we afford this type of money when our public health infrastructure is in shambles? Had we used this to bolster the public health infrastructure to manage moderate to severe cases our mortality rates would have been still lower in the second wave.

Public Health: Corporate Hospital pushed Family Physicians out but Failed to replace them.

Corporate Hospitals have pushed out the Family Physicians but size, glitz and glamour are not always effective as the Biblical tale of David vs Goliath tells us.

Goliath is a gigantic Philistine warrior with full armour, sword, and javelin, equipped with the state of the art gear for combat. He epitomizes strength backed with unlimited wealth. David on the other hand is a small lowly shepherd boy carrying a stick and a sling who dared to take on the challenge of fighting the mighty Goliath. In the ensuing contest to the amazement of all, David with his nimbleness, flexibility and adaptability, brings down the clumsy, groping, Goliath by a sharp stone thrown from his sling.

Down the ages people have assumed that Goliath, given his size and heavy armour, had the advantage in this unequal combat and David's victory over Goliath was a fluke against all odds.

Recently, Malcolm Gladwell based on published research has reinterpreted this biblical tale in his book "'David and Goliath: Underdogs, Misfits, and the Art of Battling Giants."' Gladwell affirms that we get this famous legend often wrong as we misunderstand who had the upper hand in this uneven match. Scientific and theological investigations have unravelled many fascinating facts surrounding the clash between David and Goliath.

A peer reviewed paper by Dierdee Donnelly and Patrick Morrison titled, "'Hereditary Gigantism' – the biblical Goliath and his brothers, published in Ulster Medical Journal in 2014, after meticulous study of the description of Goliath in original Hebrew theology texts and current scientific information, conclude that Goliath suffered from acromegaly caused by a tumour of the pituitary gland at the base of the brain. This condition increases the secretion of the growth hormone which leads to gigantism.

The tumour also presses on the optic nerve which carries visual images from the eyes to the brain and can lead to double vision and severe nearsightedness. Goliath is blind is evident in the biblical narrative where he has to be led by hand to the contest. The big lumbering giant is also weighed down by his cumbersome heavy armour making his movements clumsy and slow. David while no match in size but with advantage of speed and flexibility vanquished his mighty foe with a precise throw from his sling.

Gladwell says lessons from this ancient tale are applicable to big monolithic organisations. The very things which make these organizations formidable such as size, huge resources, state of the art technology, often weigh down these companies like Goliath's heavy armour and limit their vision leading to big and unexpected failures. After a period of growth, size transforms from advantage to a handicap. Conflicts of interests, absent in times of Goliath, deprives them of autonomy.

Parallels can be drawn to these dynamics in the *gigantic* heights reached by medicine and public health in recent decades. Remarkable advances in medical technology such as genomics, precision medicine, and biotechnology have transformed medicine to "'gigantic"' or "'acromegalous"' heights! The accompanying costs and challenges of sustaining technology have made individual practice give way to corporate hospitals transforming medicine from a calling to big business propped up by pharmaceutical giants.

The sheer size and *gigantic* visibility of the medico-pharmacological industry has given rise to unrealistic expectations among people that every ill has a pill. No doubt medical advances have led to remarkable improvements in health and wellness of people. But like in the case of Goliath, the vision and flexibility of this faceless growing industry has contracted and diminished. It should be a matter of concern and introspection for all. Fall of this medical giant can be catastrophic for humankind. The writing on the wall is ominous.

The response of this medical Goliath to the latest pandemic brought these limitations to the fore. Faced with a nimble, small, fast spreading, and adaptable foe in the form of SARS-CoV-2 it groped and tottered clumsily to vanquish the invisible enemy. The clumsy visionless movements of this giant trampled upon lives and livelihoods across the globe. Prolonged restrictive measures like lockdowns destroyed businesses and fractured society.

While the initial awkward and uncoordinated response in face of many unknowns was understandable, the giant failed to adapt itself to accumulating evidence. It kept on persisting with the restrictive measures for all when data indicated that the novel virus is lethal mostly for frail elderly or people with co- morbidities. Schools and educational institutions were closed and continued to be closed in many countries when evidence indicated that risks to young people and children were minimal and far less than many risks of daily life such as accidents and other endemic diseases.

Just as Goliath flung blindly at David without making any impact, the mainstay of the Covid-19 response continued to depend on blind chase of the virus by contact tracing and quarantine even when the virus silently spread through communities and these resource intensive measures did not shown to make any dent and were futile and costly during the later stages of the pandemic.

Just as a pituitary tumour keeps on growing and secretes more growth hormone the increasing size diminishing vision further, the pandemic response stimulated more technology by way of expanding vaccines for all ages including young people and children who are at minimal risk, while the nimble virus continued to adapt by way of more mutations. This frantic mass vaccination campaigns were being rolled out even in countries where every two persons out of three had recovered from natural infection as revealed by serosurveys. Research shows that natural infection confers robust immunity while same cannot be said about vaccines. Long time adverse effects, if any, of the vaccines which are under emergency use authorization are also unknown.

In this crisis, many would be missing the "'*Davids*"' of medicine, i.e., the general practitioners of a bygone era, with a stethoscope symbolic of the sling. They would wonder whether these Davids would have performed better with their flexible and customized approach, instead of the costly "'state of the art"' armour of RT-PCR and chest scans with a host of costly and useless repurposed drugs. They would also wonder whether a David would have coerced them, to get vaccinated from a growing choice of rapidly developed vaccines. The giant Goliath besides trampling on livelihoods in the mad chase for the virus continued to do all these for a disease in which 99.9% of all those who catch the virus survive.

The combat between the *giant* and the nimble virus is continuing so it would be inappropriate to predict or pass judgment on who will win or what is the right approach. Posterity will judge.

Military Lessons for Medical Leaders.

Ignoring tropical diseases in the country and blindly following ill-informed Western leads is a costly mistake.

Kurt von Hammerskin-Equord, a German general and a long-time opponent of Adolf Hitler and the Nazi regime, conceived a classification scheme for military leaders, "'I distinguish four types. There are clever, hardworking, stupid, and lazy officers. Usually two characteristics are combined. Some are clever and hardworking; their place is the General Staff. The next ones are stupid and lazy; they make up 90 percent of every army and are suited to routine duties. Anyone who is both clever and lazy is qualified for the highest leadership duties, because he possesses the mental clarity and strength of nerve necessary for difficult decisions. One must beware of anyone who is both stupid and hardworking; he must not be entrusted with any responsibility because he will always only cause damage."'

The global medical community declared war on SARS-CoV-2. The costs and collateral damage perhaps reached the scale of the earlier two great military wars. Pandemic operations on war footing call for leadership qualities of high calibre on par with that of military wars. Important insights can be obtained by analyzing the leadership styles which shaped the strategies and continue to do so in the ongoing war against the pandemic.

Unfortunately, the lead in the present war on the pandemic was taken by medical thought leaders whose lack of experience made them take draconian measures causing immense collateral harm. Experts from the West, who led the global war against the pandemic lacked battle experience as they handle few communicable diseases. However they dominate mainstream medical thinking. Medical literature published by them are read with reverence usually reserved for holy scriptures! Retractions of research based on fake data from some of their reputed journals during the pandemic make us wonder whether all along we have been worshipping false gods!

The response of these experts to the threat of the novel SARS-CoV-2 is reminiscent of the classic tale of Don Quixote and his aide Sancho Panza epitomizing deluded leadership. The Quixotic delusion such as mistaking windmills for monsters gave rise to the idiom "‘tilting at windmills"’ implying attacking imagined enemies. In management parlance it amounts to addressing issues which are unimportant or impossible to overcome. In spite of his delusions Don Quixote wins Panza's devotion and admiration.

Delusion of a highly lethal virus led to panic in the medical leadership. When leadership panics, the common people panic manifold. To be fair, this delusion of high lethality was due to limited data in the initial stages of the pandemic. Whatever figures were available were from seriously ill hospital cases. Naturally these overestimated the lethality. The highly rated journal Lancet published an early paper estimating a death rate of 20% from the novel virus.

However, a good military leader monitors information from the battlefield to calibrate his attack with changing dynamics. In the pandemic even when studies revealed that majority of infections are asymptomatic, mild and self limiting, killing less than 0.3% die of those infected - misguided efforts and resources continued to be wasted on questionable control policies.

The strategy adopted by most countries was to use restrictive measures to "‘break the chain of transmission"’ to act as speed breakers and give breathing space to overwhelmed hospital services. In military operations, this can be compared to temporary retreat to check mass casualties.

Meanwhile, vaccine development moved at great speed aided by novel gene based technology. This generated optimism of quick victory and an unrealistic target of zero cases.

Why this strategy was flawed? A good general fights a war on all fronts. This basic principle was overlooked and continued to be overlooked in the single mindedsingle-minded attack on only one front, i.e., Covid-19. When the hurly-burly is done, when the battle is lost and won we may come to the bitter truth that we lost more lives from loss of livelihoods than lives saved from Covid-19.

While the medical leaders of the West may be condoned for their naivety as most have not done real battle with communicable diseases, the acts of omissions and commissions of our own advisers amount to a Himalayan blunder. The burden and mortality from any of our endemic diseases are much higher than Covid-19. We should have realized that given the sheer size of our population and its density off the shelf "‘one size fits all"’ solutions from the West will not work.

The elephant in the room presently was our already very high level of population level immunity. The fourth round of serosurvey undertaken by Indian Council of Medical Research in June 2021 revealed country wide seropositivity of 67% which translates to 93 crores Indians having antibodies to SARS-CoV-2. This has resulted mostly from widespread community transmission of natural infection, as the vaccination coverage during this study was less than 5%.

According to well established principles of immunology having acquired natural infection which may be symptomatic or asymptomatic confers robust immunity better than any vaccine. This was also repeatedly confirmed by ongoing studies across the globe. A study from Israel established that natural infection gives 13 times stronger immunity than that conferred by vaccination. Another important point in our favour was that the second wave in our country which was more than four times more massive and widespread than the first wave was due to the delta variant. Having faced its havoc, our population earned herd immunity the hard way.

If we had followed the science, we may have paused to think whether it will serve any purpose to roll out mass vaccination in such a population at huge cost and resources. A good general would have conserved his heavy artillery in such a situation. We too may have considered focused vaccination in high risk groups instead of mass indiscriminate vaccination. The Chinese warrior philosopher Sun Tzu in his Art of War, stated *"'...those who are not thoroughly aware of the disadvantages in the use of arms cannot be thoroughly aware of the advantages in the use of arms."'* Vaccines are heavy artillery with us now. We should know both their disadvantages (mostly unknown, particularly long termlong-term effects) as well as their advantages and use them judiciously like a good general who conserves firepower.

Lastly, it is high time our medical decision makers and researchers stopped imitating the West blindly. We should take full advantage of the research opportunities provided by the vast variety of diseases prevalent in our country. As one of the founder fathers of the London School of Tropical Medicine, Sir Patrick Manson said more than a century ago, "'The tropical practitioner enjoys opportunities for original research and discovery far superior in novelty and interest to those at the command of his fellow inquirer in the well-worked field of European and American research."' These words from the great master should inspire our researchers. If medical researchers from developing countries do not take the lead in tropical medicine, minor ailments of affluence will get more priority than major ailments of poverty. Failure to seize the opportunity will firmly establish the era of "'Medical Imperialism"' giving rise to a new world order replacing arms race with "'pharma race."' In this race the poor countries with their neglected tropical diseases will be left far behind.

Mysterious "'Fever"' a bigger challenge than Covid

A large number of cases were reported among children in Firozabad, a city with a population of over 6 lakhs near Agra and known for its glass making industry

Post monsoons, 11 districts in Uttar Pradesh (UP) were in the grip of suspected Dengue and other fevers. The other suspected causes of fevers in these districts were scrub typhus, leptospirosis, Japanese Encephalitis (JE) which is caused by a virus, and other viral encephalitis. Even malaria or typhoid, endemic in large parts of India could have added to the numbers.

Firozabad in UP was in the centre of this outbreak of "'mysterious fever"' among children. It is a city with a population of over 6 lakhs near Agra famous for its glassmaking industry. The population density is over 1000 per km^2 more than twice the national population density. The city is on the national highway which makes it an important stopover for passing transport vehicles. The district includes a large rural belt with to and fro rural-urban movement of people in search of occupation. These create an ideal environment for spread of febrile illnesses from this epicentre to other parts of the State.

The spate of febrile illnesses hit hard in the region. There was confusion and chaos. There were reports of people fleeing from entire village as many, mostly children and young people died from "'mysterious fever."'

According to media reports thousands of people in Firozabad district were bedridden with fever at home and hospital. In a short period there were 71 reported deaths of which, tragically, 52 were among children. Out of a meagre 185 samples tested, 73 were positive for dengue, 28 for scrub typhus and one for Japanese Encephalitis.

In the eighteenth century, when being told that her French subjects had no bread, Marie-Antoinette, the Queen of France supposedly sniffed, "'Qu'ils mangent de la brioche"'—"'Let them eat cake."' With that callous remark, the queen became a hated symbol of the decadent monarchy oblivious to the poor conditions in which many of her subjects lived while she lived decadently.

We are experiencing the same ethos among the health policy makers. Here we were with one of the largest states in the country, in the grip of a "'mysterious fever"' which was killing mostly children and young people and all our resources were deployed in mass vaccination for Covid-19 which rarely kills children and young people and Quixotically preparing for the paediatric third wave. To add to the irony, vaccine trials for Covid-19 was being conducted among children with unholy haste. Schools continued to remain closed ostensibly to protect children from a "'lethal"' virus. The panic among parents was sustained so that many rush for a vaccine for their children before they go back to school.

UP health officials confirmed this thought process in a statement that with increasing cases of this "'mysterious disease"' the situation was fast turning Covid like. What an amateurish comparison! With so many deaths among children and young people from this "'mysterious fever,"' only 185 samples had been tested after a month into this outbreak, to identify the "'mysterious illness"' as compared to lakhs of RT-PCR tests to detect Covid-19 which were done every day on asymptomatic people young and old.

Post monsoons, dengue is a major public health problem in our country, year after year. It is a leading cause of hospitalization and death among children and young people. Death rate can vary from 2% - 20% depending on the severity and access to early diagnosis and management. The dreaded dengue hemorrhagic fever with severe fall in platelets and bleeding can be fatal.

The dengue virus is transmitted by bite of aedes mosquitoes which thrive in artificial water containers. The mosquito, also known as the tiger mosquito is a day biter. There are four serotypes of the virus and previous infection with one serotype does not protect against subsequent infection by a different serotype - in fact this sequential infection with different serotypes makes a person more vulnerable to the dreaded dengue hemorrhagic syndrome.

The second suspect for this "'mysterious illness"' was scrub typhus with 28 confirmed cases out of the 185 samples tested. This is caused by rickettsia, a small bacterium, named after Howard Ricketts, the American pathologist who died of it after discovering it. Scrub typhus is transmitted by bite of mites which thrive in grassy soils. Post monsoons these grassy "'mite islands"' expand. The cycle of transmission continues in nature between mites and rodents. Children playing on grassy terrain and campers are accidental victims. Scrub typhus is treated with antibiotics like tetracycline. When treated early, the mortality is 1.6%. In untreated cases the mortality can be 30-35%.

Japanese Encephalitis is a viral infection which can affect the central nervous system. It is transmitted by culex mosquitoes which breed in rice fields. The natural cycle is between mosquitoes and pigs or other animals like cattle and in birds and poultry. The animal and bird hosts do not themselves suffer from the illness (except horses), but act as amplifier hosts, i.e. the virus multiplies in them. Mostly the infection do not cause symptoms but can be fatal in children and young adults with a case fatality rate of 20% to 40%. Neurological deficits in survivors are common. Vaccine for JE is available but not promoted with the same gusto as for Covid-19.

Other diseases such as malaria and typhoid are other unfinished agenda in our country. Malaria while treatable, it can cause rapid deterioration in some cases where fatality can reach 20% even with treatment. Typhoid has a fatality rate between 1% to 4% with treatment, while without treatment the fatality rate can be as high as 10% to 30%. Children and young adults between 5 years to 19 years have the highest incidence.

Leptospirosis is also on the suspected list of probable cause of fevers. It is again an infection which spreads from waste water contaminated by urine of animals which carry the bacterial spirochetes. While it can be treated with antibiotics like penicillin death rates can vary from 5% to 30% depending on diagnostic and treatment facilities. It is common after monsoons due to water logging through which people may wade and the organisms may enter through skin abrasions or cuts.

Untreated Covid-19 has a mortality rate of 0.3% across all age groups globally and less than 0.1% in India. In children and young adults the mortality is far lower than 0.05%. With such low death rate even in the natural course of the infection it is quite difficult to evaluate impact of any therapeutic or preventive intervention.

The science and art of public health demands that scarce resources should be allocated to diseases with higher public health burden. This is determined by the death rates and potential years of life lost. From above comparative data it would be evident that all the potential causes of "‘mysterious fever"’ which created havoc in districts of Uttar Pradesh have far higher death rates and potential years of life lost as they all predominantly affect children and young people.

Offering mass vaccinations against Covid-19 to populations in such predicaments is tantamount to asking them to eat cake when they cannot afford bread!

As Professor Martin Kulldorff, a leading epidemiologist from Harvard University said on the mismanagement during the pandemic,"’We have to go back to the basic principles of public health that was thrown out the window a year ago. It’s not one disease, public health is about all the diseases, and all the collateral damage."'

Regrettably, "'following the science"' was lip service in the pandemic. In an editorial in the British Medical Journal, "'Covid-19: politicisation, "'corruption"' and suppression of Science,"' Abbasi poignantly states, "'The stakes are high for politicians, scientific advisers, and government appointees. Their careers and bank balances may hinge on the decisions that they make. But they have a higher responsibility and duty to the public. Science is a public good... When good science is suppressed, people die."'"'

Preparing for the next pandemic: take lessons from cricket.

Fast pitches can make even average bowlers look deadly. Similarly, SARS-CoV-2 was deadly on Western pitches where an ageing and obese population with unhealthy lifestyles was an easy prey.

Pandemics are fought on war footing. A lot goes into the preparation for war. Most of it is behind the scenes and unexciting. An old dictum, "'The more you sweat in peace, the less you bleed in war,"' sums it up. How does one go about this unglamorous preparation?

Napoleon, one of the greatest military strategists in history, was defeated by the Duke of Wellington at Waterloo bringing an end to the Napoleonic era of European history. What preparations let to this historic victory?

According to the Duke, who was a graduate of Eton College, a keen cricketer, and Commander in Chief of the British and Allied Armies at Waterloo, "'The battle of Waterloo was won on the playing fields of Eton."' Well, the preparation for war need not be unglamorous after all!

Like the Duke of Wellington, the world can borrow strategies from the game of cricket to prepare for war against the next pandemic. Failure teaches us more than success. The strategic blunders committed during the current pandemic can provide lessons for planning for the next disaster.

A new bowler pushes the batting side on the back foot ripping through the batting order with the batsmen ducking and removing their eyes from the ball. The novel coronavirus too created havoc globally and the world ducked. In the chaos and anarchy, unprecedented measures were implemented fracturing society and destroying the economy. The captains driving leading medical consensus took their eyes off the ball. In their haste and arrogance they ignored the few feeble voices of umpires who raised concerns that such measures were unconstitutional and violation of human rights. While China, which never plays cricket in any case, locked down a single district, other countries went for nationwide lockdowns at short notice driving the poor and marginalized to misery. Most other countries too ceased to play cricket.

The captains in this pandemic failed to read the pitches in different countries. Bowlers in cricket, however furious and fast do not have the same impact on all pitches. On English pitches they may be fast and deadly, turning out to be more benign on slower Indian pitches.

The virus too encountered different pitches at different places. Fast pitches can make even average bowlers appear deadly. Similarly, the novel coronavirus was deadly on Western pitches while much less so in African and Asian continents. Captains in different countries could have customized country-specific strategies. They instead went for "'one-size-fits-all"' restrictive and harsh measures.

The novel virus ran through the aged population of the West, particularly the vulnerable in nursing homes. A large proportion of deaths occurred in people in their eighties with co-morbidities. As the captains of strategy had taken their eyes off the ball, lack of plans to protect this vulnerable group caused severe disease and deaths overwhelming the health services and aggravating the global panic. Death rates from these pitches provided inputs for mathematical models predicting global catastrophe. Amongst this anarchy, policy makers took vital decisions affecting millions of lives and livelihoods.

In addition to higher age, population in the West have three times higher rates of obesity compared to the East. Obesity, is a risk factor for severe disease and death.

The virus had less impact on the leaner and younger populations of the African and Asian countries. This difference stares one on the face on the scoreboard on the "'Worldometer."' Few outliers give further insights. Japan has one of the oldest populations. Paradoxically, it has a far lower death rate. The reason may be much leaner population compared to the West – the proportion of people in Japan who are overweight is 25% compared to European and American population where it is around 60%. The other paradox is Brazil. It is a fast growing economy, with a comparatively younger population. Still it is experiencing high severity and deaths from the pandemic. Almost 60% of Brazilians are overweight. Obesity is turning out to be a bigger risk factor than age.

Overlooking these patterns, leaders and policy makers of most nations gave the impression of fumbling captains making hasty decisions on being forced to play on unpredictable pitches. No attempt was made by nations particularly from Asian and African continents to make an assessment of local conditions, including demographics and population profiles.

The Achilles heel in Asian countries like India, is lack of fielders, poor field placement and lack of scoreboards, i.e., a proper disease surveillance system, for most endemic diseases. Meagre available resources and infrastructure are concentrated in urban areas. The second wave in India revealed these fault lines. Rather than the lethality of the virus (in India the infection fatality rate from Covid-19 is0.1% compared to global figure of 0.3%), these limitations caused a large number of preventable deaths.

How do we prepare for future pandemics? The present pandemic indicates that lifestyle factors such as obesity are as important to reduce severity and deaths from acute communicable diseases as they are for chronic diseases. This pandemic is a wakeup call not only for the Western countries but also for fast growing economies in Asia and Africa where unhealthy life styles are catching up fast. These factors damage the pitch and could again spell disaster in case of future emerging pathogens and pandemics. Development of vaccines takes time and do not afford full proof protection as is becoming evident. Even with helmets and body guards, players can get injured due to lack of practice and damaged pitches.

Countries like India have to improve its field placement. Long term planning should address the rural urban disparities in public health infrastructure. The state needs to invest more in public health. It also needs a good scoreboard i.e. a disease surveillance and monitoring system. The Covid-19 template of monitoring and surveillance can be extended to our endemic communicable diseases such as dengue, scrub typhus, typhoid, Japanese Encephalitis, malaria and others. Private insurance and corporate model of health care, as is being increasingly adopted involves an ever increasing number of stakeholders with their own vested interests. A noble game like cricket fell from grace at times due to high stakes and incidents of match-fixing. We need to insulate the noble profession from increasing conflicts of interest and a similar fate.

And of course, Americans need to play a little cricket too besides baseball. There are no pitches in baseball which may perhaps explain the limited perspectives of American thought leaders in this pandemic which acted as bellwether for the world.

Public Health: Doctors losing out to pharma and tech companies.

Commercial and political interests have overshadowed medicine and doctors' autonomy has been eroded significantly

Miyamoto Musashi, the Japanese swordsman, philosopher and strategist born in the 16th century, refined a two sword technique, naming it "two heavens as one," or "One School - Two Swords, *"Nito Ichi Ryu."* This is the teaching of the school founded by this great Samurai. He stresses the correct choice of using the long and short swords. The best use of the short or companion sword is in a confined space or when engaged in hand to hand combat. The long sword can be used judiciously in all situations.

Using this analogy in the fight against disease, the short or companion sword for the physician is symbolized by the stethoscope and the doctor's clinical skills. The long sword can be compared with costly and state of the art investigations and application of medical technology. Increasingly, the use of this long sword at the cost of the short sword, with good intentions no doubt, is alienating the patient and escalating the cost of medical care.

Young doctors out of medical schools are fascinated by technology or the long glittery sword. Rightly so, the marvels of modern medicine are often miraculous. However, for majority of human ills, the short sword, wielded with the art of medicine offers better outcomes improving the doctor-patient relationship. It is also cost-effective.

The reality hit me years ago when the long sword was not very long either. As a young doctor in the military posted in a remote field station in northeast India, I would see my patients, mostly young soldiers, in the morning before rushing to the nearby military hospital to learn from "interesting cases" from specialist doctors. Once while taking a leisurely stroll in the evening in civil clothes, I saw a queue in front of my office. I enquired from the last man in the queue the reason. I was informed that "doctor sahib" is seeing patients. I was surprised. I told him that the doctor comes in the morning not in the evening. I was informed in hushed tones that the doctor who comes in the morning is no good while the one who comes in the evening is excellent.

Highly curious by now, I tiptoed to the window and looked inside. It was a humbling experience. My medical assistant was attending to the patients and talking with them in their mother tongue. He was explaining to them my illegible notes. In the remote area away from family and friends, the medical assistant was the friend, philosopher and guide. My technical knowledge or the "long sword" was no match for his "short sword." While I was using the long sword in the morning he was complementing it with the short sword in the evening. I realized that to become a consummate physician, I should not abandon the use of the short sword in my eagerness to master the potentials of the "long sword."

The "consummate doctor" is rare in the current environment. This doctor is equally skilled in making a diagnosis as in customizing treatment to each patients' and families' needs, understanding that the human connection is vital to establish rapport and contributes to compliance and cure.

History taking was an art which refined communication skills. This combined with examining the patient in person cemented the doctor-patient relationship. The practice of medicine was patient-centric.

With technological advances, the length of the long sword is ever increasing, making it unwieldy. While these advances make real time diagnosis feasible, the modern physician is, literally, losing touch with the patient, with adverse impact on the doctor-patient relationship.

Like swordsmanship of a past era, medicine too started as an art. In both the encounters were close and intimate. The short sword dominated both in combat and in medicine.

The "art of combat" gave way to the "science of combat" escalating to nuclear, chemical and biological warfare. Combat became blunt and artless, accompanied with more collateral damages. In all modern wars, civilian casualties are colossal. The nuclear holocaust of Hiroshima and Nagasaki which ended the Second World War stands testimony to the potential for catastrophe when the long sword grows unchecked and assumes nuclear properties. Moderation by artful use of the short sword is needed to save humanity from extinction. Easier said than done. The arms race have molded both the short and long swords into a single sword of Damocles hanging over us threatening extinction of life on earth. Powerful and invisible forces have drastically curbed the autonomy of the simple soldier. He no longer has the option of choosing the swords. Commercial interests, political influence and the arms trade have destroyed the art of war.

Similar crises of identify is facing medicine today. It is one of the oldest arts but the youngest science, softer than the hard sciences, rich in possibility and promise says Siddhartha Mukherjee in his book, "The Laws of Medicine - Field Notes from an Uncertain Science." Regrettably, it too is becoming increasingly commercialized. Like in combat, so in medicine, commercial interests, political influence and pharmaceutical companies are increasingly restricting the autonomy of doctors. Diseases and pandemics are seen as opportunities to follow Winston Churchill's dictum, "Never let a good crisis go to waste."

The world is facing a double challenge today. Arms race and pharma race. Both need speed-breakers and traffic signals. Humanity should introspect in advance rather than after a catastrophe like the nuclear holocaust in Hiroshima and

Nagasaki which made Albert Einstein regret his suggestions on atomic research, with the words, "Woe is me."

The world is facing a dilemma due to the break neck speed at which technology has progressed. It is not "Doctors' Dilemma" like in an era when medicine was still an art. Autonomy and decision making of doctors have diluted long ago. The already complex field of medicine has become more complex to the point of being incomprehensive. The level of noise can make complex decisions difficult if not impossible. It has become "People's Dilemma."

The present mRNA technology for vaccines is remarkable and has the potential of being a game changer in our fight against disease and pandemics. But like all powerful technologies, it should be used with caution. There are some reports of vaccines manufactured by this technology causing myocarditis (an inflammation of heart muscle), particularly in young people. One of the inventors of this technology has expressed a word of caution in mass scale use of this technology.

Regrettably, the scientific community has become polarized on the issue at a time when all opposing views should be carefully examined and debated. In the heady excitement of the new technology the scientific and political consensus is moving at breakneck speed ignoring all speed-breakers and traffic signals like a reckless teenager driving his first car. One only can pray that there is no crash down the road.

Global Response to Covid-19 pandemic has been amateurish; Complex issues need many thinking hats.

Panic, fear and irrational behaviour allowed greed to exploit the pandemic. We have lessons to learn from the way we dealt with Covid

The global response to the current pandemic has been amateurish from the very beginning. Lockdowns, school closures and physical distancing were based on a school computer project of a 14 year old school student in the USA, daughter of a computer scientist. It overlooked that humans are not inert computer units but social beings. Similarly, study of efficacy of masks was first done on hamsters under laboratory conditions overlooking that humans do not behave like hamsters inside or outside the lab! Subsequent randomized trials, in Denmark and Bangladesh on efficacy of masks, thankfully in humans this time, revealed negligent to very modest impact.

Covid-19 is not as simple as it looks, or, counter intuitively, a simple problem was turned into a complex one.

Edward de Bono, a Maltese physician, and a multifaceted personality, proposed that for finding solutions to complex issues, the technique of Six Thinking Hats can contribute immensely in developing a blueprint free from biases of information, optimism, pessimism, emotions, at the same time making way for creative solutions and seeing the big picture.

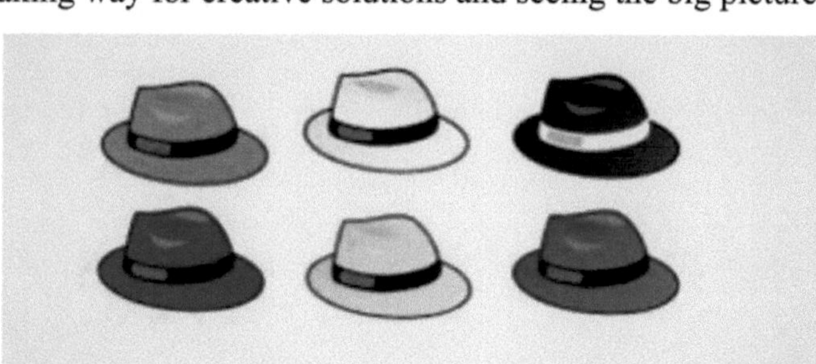

A "‘thinking hat"’ is symbolic of thinking without falling in love with your idea, as hats can be replaced. Bono proposed giving a colour to each of the hats encompassing the range of human thoughts and emotions. The colours are; white, red, yellow, black, green and blue.

The "‘White Hat"’ signifies the hard facts and figures on which sound decisions are taken. The "‘Red Hat"’ demands the soft skills of knowing the emotions such as fear, hope, beliefs, attitudes and faith which may be realistic, and often unrealistic; the "‘Yellow Hat"’ like sunshine denotes optimism which may be based on facts and sometimes not; the "‘Black Hat"’ does the role of the devil's advocate proposing caution and to consider the downside of any policy; the "‘Green Hat"’ symbolizing new growth dwells on innovative solutions and finally "‘The Blue Hat"’ looks at the big picture and ensures all hats are used.

In the covid pandemic, rakish cowboys wearing hats of a single colour hijacked issues and shot down people wearing other hats. The gullible public, the majority, in most countries, too numbed to think clearly, accepted whatever hats were thrust on their heads. Most of these were red hats of emotions - fear, panic and anxiety. Cowed into submission they were happy hunting ground for exploiters wearing the red hat of greed, be it politicians, market forces or career scientists.

Let us address the pandemic using all six hats. First the white hat, the hard data. Latest pooled data confirms that the initial estimates of lethality were highly exaggerated, as most who died in the West were around 80 years with co-morbidities. Only 6% of the reported Covid-19 deaths were solely due to the virus. Subsequent research attribute much lower lethality to the virus. The table shows the age wise survival rates by researchers from Stanford University.

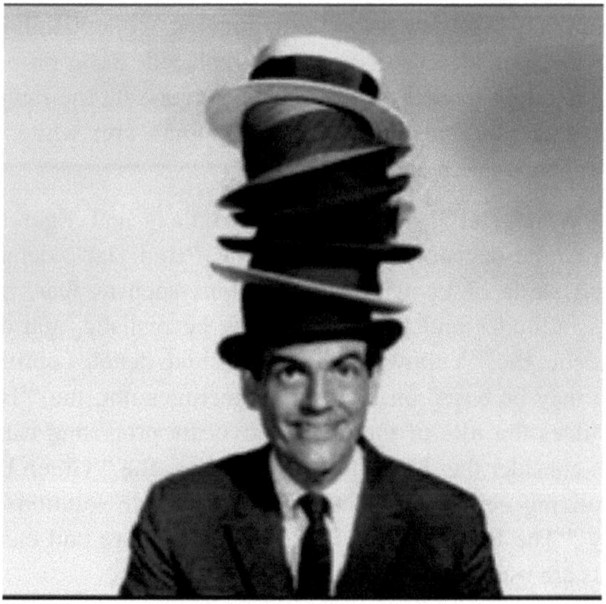

Age wise survival rates after Covid

Source https://opentheword.org/2021/08/30/survival-rates-after-contracting-covid/

Age in Years	Survival Rate
0 – 19	99.9973%
20 – 29	99.986%
30 – 39	99.969%
40 – 49	99.918%
50 – 59	99.73%
60 – 69	99. 41%
70 +	97.6%
70 + (in care Home)	94. 5%

From this white paper...er...white hat it is evident that the risk of dying from Covid-19 for children and young people is negligible. This is very important for policy since a recent paper in Toxicology Reports titled, "'Why are we vaccinating children against Covid-19,"' concludes that deaths from Covid-19 in children are negligible, but post vaccination deaths in children are not negligible. Particular concerns have been raised in the paper about the spike protein of the vaccine, which have been found in different organs, and the uncertain long- term effects, - "'black hat"' thinking. These concerns are serious as data for England and Wales from 01 May 2021 until 17 September show excess deaths ranging from 16% to 47% above expected levels, in 15-19 year15–19-year males, coincident with the roll out of the vaccine in this age group. (https://www.hartgroup.org/recent-deaths-in-young-people-in-england-and-wales/). The black hat is getting blacker.

Let us move to the red hat, the emotions. The red hat on people evoked emotions of fear and panic, concerns that their children will fall prey to the virus. The red hat on exploiters promoted greed pushing for mass vaccination of children. Both these red hats, the panic and the greed should be checked by the white and black hats.

What about the yellow hat? Yellow hat thinking is influenced by perceptions. For those who use white hat i.e. data extensively to assess risks and benefits, the low mortality is a cause for optimism. For those who succumb to propaganda without looking at the data, blind faith in the vaccine brings optimism. Regrettably this is the majority creating a happy hunting ground for vested interests. "'Expert"' narrative fuelled this faith in vaccines as the saviour of humankind. Waiting for the vaccine justified prolonged lockdowns and associated misery. The inflated estimates of lethality of the virus were not corrected in people's mind leading to a sort of "'medical stampede"' during the second wave in India whereby majority of people who had Rt-PCR positive results but were having mild to no symptoms rushed to hospitals overwhelming the system and depriving serious cases of much needed beds and oxygen. If the white hat been used judiciously from the beginning this "'stampede"' could have been avoided saving many lives.

After the vaccine roll out in many countries, we have more data for "'white hat thinking"' which should guide policy. A paper in the European Journal of Epidemiology is sobering. The study published online on 30 September 2021, titled, "'Increases in Covid-19 are unrelated to levels of vaccination across 68 countries and 2947 counties in the United States,"' concludes that vaccines should be offered with humility and respect without stigmatizing (excessive use of the red hat), as mass vaccination does not seem to check transmission. A bit of black hat there.

Well, other studies gives us reason to don the yellow hat, particularly in our country. Studies from Israel among others, have established that recovery from natural infections gives 13 times more robust immunity compared to vaccines. Solid white hat data. The serosurvey in June 2021 by ICMR had brought out that almost 70% Indians and considerable number of children had recovered from the infection and have acquired natural immunity. By any standard, this amounts to herd immunity of the population. So even without the mass vaccination rollout, there was no chance of the dreaded third wave.

What role did the creative green hat driving innovation, play in this pandemic? A laudable one. It brought new technology in vaccine development paving the way for vaccine development for other diseases. However, like a strong force, it should be tempered with the remaining five hats. Just because a technology has been developed it should not be used indiscriminately. It can harm as emerging signals from the data (white hat) indicate.

And lastly the green hat, seeing the big picture. The green hat should balance all the hats equitably and change hats according to the situation and region. No one hat should get stuck indefinitely on our head. Presently the role of the green hat is to distribute a lot of white hats (data) and yellow hats (optimism based on data), and some black hat too (regarding the efficacy/harm of vaccines, based on white hat driven data). And of course, the major role is to remove the red hats among the population who are still in panic mode and the red hat of "'greed"' among the exploiters which include politicians, career scientists and market forces.

Conflicting claims on efficacy of masks

Masks have been 80% effective in stopping the spread of coronavirus, says the CDC. Other medical researches show a more modest efficacy of 11% or no efficacy at all

In social interactions nuanced deviations from the truth or "'pro-social lies"' can occasionally tide over a thorny situation. Extending this to science can bring about its nemesis. And if practiced by haloed scientific institutions these can result in irreparable harm to their credibility and reputation.

During the pandemic such deviations from evidence based practice became rather too frequent on the part of reputable institutions like the Centre for Disease Control (CDC), Atlanta, USA, the United States Food and Drug Administration (FDA), and others. Misinformation from esteemed institutions which had been acknowledged as the final authority by scientists, researchers, and the general public, can have devastatingly adverse impact on the current and future pandemics. It can lead to irreparable erosion of trust among the general public in science and scientific institutions, and also cause dismay and disillusionment, if not a little embarrassment, among practicing researchers. These misguiding signals also have the potential to push research priorities down the wrong path.

In English art and literature, Shakespeare, or the Bard, as he was known, is said to have captured the whole gamut of the human experience including deceit, greed, and pathos, using melodrama to appeal to the emotion of the masses. In Julius Caesar, one of his well known tragedies, Caesar's last words were, "'Et tu, Brute, Than fall Caesar"' which translates to "'You too, Brutus, than fall Caesar"' as Caesar's assassins included his best and trusted friend Brutus.

Indian mainstream art and culture too captures this vast canvas through current medium of mass entertainment, the movies. A song in a classic Hindi movie captures the current state of affairs in medical science. In this song there are many allegories to this situation. For instance, there is a stanza which goes, *"'Majdhaar Mai Naiyya Dole, to Majhi Paar Lagaye, Majhi Jo Nao Duboye Ushe Kaun Bachai..."'* which translates to *"'In the midstream, when the boat is wobbling, the boatman saves it from going down, but when the boatman himself sinks the boat, who will save it."'*

The pandemic exposed the cracks in our public health and regulatory systems. USA being the bellwether of global trends misinformation and misdemeanours on part of those entrusted to safeguard public health and ensure safety of interventions for controlling pandemics is cause for great concern and a threat to humanity.

During the pandemic, the CDC Director tweeted that masks cut down transmission of the novel coronavirus by 80%. This statement, which flies in the face of evidence, coming from the CDC director did immense harm to the credibility of this august institution. CDC Atlanta used to be the last word in public health protocols and this highly inaccurate statement had the potential to undermine the trust of public health professionals in the CDC. Far lesser deviations from the truth by lesser mortals are labelled as "'fake news"' by the mainstream consensus and censored.

The scientific evidence of protection by masks is that cloth masks do not check transmission of the virus and surgical masks offer very modest protection to the tune of 11%. A Danish Randomized Controlled Mask Study did not find any benefit of using surgical masks while a very large Cluster Randomized Mask Study from Bangladesh found that cloth masks offered no protection while surgical masks reduced transmission by mere 11%.

Such misinformation can be hazardous. The misleading statement of 80% efficacy by masks could lull many into a false sense of security. Overestimating the protection offered, most may neglect other safe behaviour such as the three ‘Cs,’ i.e. avoid closed spaces, crowds and close contacts. This can be hazardous particularly for the old and vulnerable.

Masks not used properly can be extremely hazardous. In hot humid weather sweat and saliva can wet the masks within a couple of hours providing ideal soil for growth of other pathogens and fungi more virulent than the novel coronavirus. A hypothesis can be proposed that the high incidence of mucormycosis or black fungi during the second wave in hot and humid summer of India might have been due to improperly used soiled masks besides use of steroids and underlying diabetes. This is a topic for research which was never explored. This may have been due to the belief that masks are holy and sacrosanct the way they were advocated by people in high places such as the Director of CDC without any evidence, rather against all evidence.

Another clumsy and amateurish action by CDC was the propaganda that vaccine induced immunity was superior to immunity after recovery from natural infection based on a highly flawed study. This study was an observations one on a sample of just 89 unrepresentative patients in various hospitals and has been criticised severely by serious researchers. On the other hand, real world studies on very large sample sizes in Israel and Cleveland Clinic, USA among others, have established beyond reasonable doubt that immunity after natural infection confers at least 13 times more robust immunity compared to vaccine induced immunity. The CDC had to eat its words later, when events overtook the false narrative, and had to concede that natural immunity was superior to vaccine induced immunity.

The FDA too was complicit in acts of omission if not commission. According to an investigative article in the prestigious British Medical Journal (BMJ), there were gross irregularities in one of the centres conducting the Pfizer vaccine trials. The director of this centre reported the sloppy quality control during the vaccine trials such as untrained vaccinators, poor follow up of adverse events, unblended participants and other lapses to the FDA. This regulatory body even on being informed about these lapses did not take any action. To add insult to injury, the whistleblower was summarily sacked by her employers.

Such acts of omissions and commissions by august bodies like the CDC and regulatory authorities like the FDA echoes the pathos of the Bard and that in the classic music song questioning who will save us from drowning if the boatman himself sinks the boat. "'Et tu CDC, Et tu FDA, than fall Science!'" or "'*Majhi Jo Nao Duboye Ushe Kaun Bachai...*'"

If Omicron is the second new ball, it is unlikely to cause much damage because the pitch has slowed.

If the new variant of the coronavirus was the second new ball in a Test match, it was unlikely to do much damage because the pitch had slowed and there was no grass.

The strategy to check the current covid-19 pandemic which started like a limited- overs cricket match seamlessly took the form of a test match due to the crisis becoming protracted. The initial promise was a limited two to three weeks lockdown in most countries. This was ostensibly to "'"flatten-the-curve"'" and "'"break the chain"'" of transmission, allowing time to boost up the health infrastructure and prevent them from getting overwhelmed. This expected short term manoeuvre turned into long term restrictions in most countries in anticipation of availability of vaccine round the corner. The pandemic threatened to settle into the longest version of the game with arrival of the "'"second new ball"'", the Omicron variant of the novel coronavirus.

The first new ball was the Delta variant with perceived nip and pace. The panic of this first new ball led to high fatalities as large number of asymptomatic and mild cases scrambled for admission to hospitals in a sort of "'"medical stampede."'" The associated chaos and anarchy affected care of those patients who really needed it. This contributed to large number of fatalities some of which could have been prevented had the pandemic been managed according to the principles of public health.

To avoid making the same strategic blunders with the arrival of the second new ball, the Omnicron variant, we should take a hard look not only at the new ball but also on the pitch which influences the swing and nip of the new ball. In the last days of the test match the pitch loses grass and pace. Population too develop a very high level of herd immunity predominantly after recovery from natural infection which renders a more robust and long lasting immunity.

Viruses to survive follow nature's laws of adaptation - Darwin's Law. These adaptations are by way of mutations, natural phenomena, not new, due to errors during replication, and occasionally due to selection pressure, like mass vaccination during a pandemic. According to principles of successful parasitism, this adaptation is beneficial to both the virus and humans. Errors that make the virus fittest for survival propagate while others lose out due to laws of natural selection. Lethal or virulent strains perish with the victim leading to a dead end infection. Less virulent strains which do not kill but cause symptoms also do not go far because patients resort to self isolation. Thousands of such mutations have already occurred with the novel coronavirus, majority of them going undetected.

The mutant strains, which survive and go far, are the least virulent ones which do not kill the host and cause very mild symptoms, if any. People infected with such benign variants will mingle with other and transmit these mutants wide and far. The high contagiousness does not translate to high lethality directly. The new mutant Omnicron is following the Darwin's law of natural selection perfectly. From reports so far, it causes very mild self limiting symptoms.

It is very important therefore, not to raise the panic button at every subsequent variant, which by the laws of natural selection would tend to be more benign, by sealing borders and imposing quarantines and lockdowns, measures which did not achieve any interruption of transmission of earlier less contagious variants. These mistakes will raise fear and anxiety among people leading to a medical stampede where asymtomatic patients fill up the hospital beds and drain medical resources depriving the severe cases much needed management.

With the bulk of the Indian population having immunity from natural infection which always give more robust and more long lasting immunity compared to vaccine immunity, as the body's immune system and memory and T cells are exposed to the whole virus for 10-15 days compared to vaccine induced immunity which is directed only at the spike protein (where 30 mutations have taken place), the Omnicron and subsequent mutants would not pose a problem in the country. On the other hand, due to their higher infectivity coupled with negligible lethality, they may raise the population level immunity still higher applying full brakes to the pandemic which has already entered the endemic state in India, bringing it to a dead halt.

Historically, natural infections even after decades give long lasting immunity even without vaccination. This has happened with H1N1 pandemic in 2009 when people over 60 had milder impact compared to the young

Immunity to the novel coronavirus too shows cross immunity from infection from previous SARS infection. People exposed to SARS-CoV-1 17 years ago show strong T-cell immunity to the SARS-CoV-2 according to published research.

Keeping all these factors in mind, Omnicron and subsequent variants may achieve at population level what any ideal vaccine should achieve, i.e. raising the herd immunity without causing fatalities or hospitalization. Chasing such a mild variant with huge resources is akin to chasing the common cold. Only the moderate to severe cases should be monitored leaving the asymptomatic cases alone.

Last but not the least, stakeholders with conflicts of interests including pharmaceutical industry, private players, politicians and career scientists should be "'quarantined.'" This will promote good science and lead humanity back to sanity. Anything short of this will result in a wild goose chase of zero covid cases even when new variants cause zero deaths leading to huge economic and social setbacks.

The Covid-19 Chess Game: Are we seeing all the pieces and their combinations on the board?

While the clinician sees only one piece at a time, the epidemiologist sees all the pieces and their combinations which is essential to tackle public health problems.

One of my favourite methods of teaching epidemiology is to compare this fascinating field with the game of chess. While a clinician treating individual patients sees a disease problem in piecemeal, an epidemiologist sees the big picture.

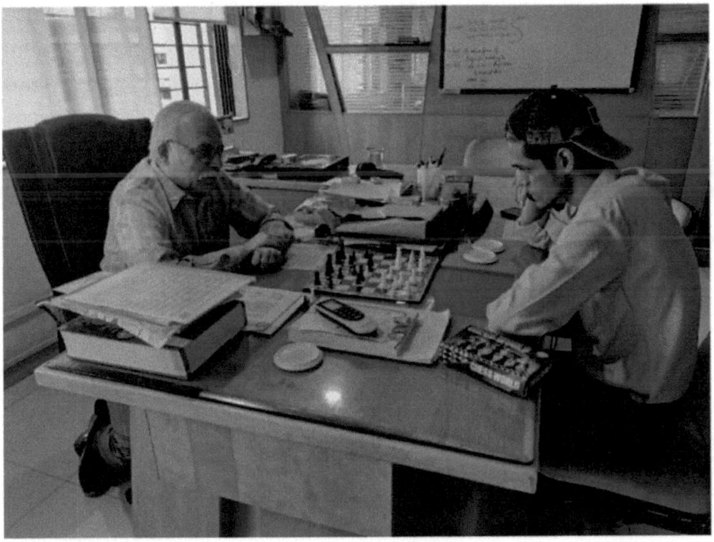

In chess, the beginner gets fascinated with the queen and neglects the other pieces. A good player sees all the chess pieces and also the combinations of the pieces with each other. A novice who focuses only on the queen loses easily to an experienced player. In chess, seeing one's own pieces as well as the opponent's pieces and their relationships to each other is important to win.

The Covid-19 virus was the queen on the chess board for the past two years. Self styled experts like novice players had their vision firmly focused on it oblivious to the other pieces and their combinations on the chess board on which the Covid-19 chess game continued to be played. From the early phase itself, i.e. May 2020, black represented by the Asian and African countries, was winning. This lead continues throughout the pandemic..

A rapid look at the data showing deaths per million population 03 May 2020 and on 12 Dec 2021 from a sample of Western, Asian and African countries will make this apparent [Tables 1 – 3].

Western countries have better hygiene and sanitation with much lower population density than most Asian and African Countries, still they had the hi. Most African and South Asian countries have very high population densities with a large part of their population staying in slums where "'physical distancing"' and "'hand washing"' the measures promoted to control spread of Covid-19 is just not feasible. Also the black side of the board has many times less vaccination cover than the white.

The same pattern can be observed in almost all the countries in Africa and South Asia shown in Tables. Western countries which can indulge in the privilege of physical distancing and frequent hand washing and with much higher vaccination coverage, are, throughout the pandemic, having many times more fatalities from Covid-19 than the crowded and unhygienic populations of South Asian and African countries with very low vaccination coverage.

Table 1. Deaths from Covid-19 in some Western Countries

Country	Deaths/IM Population 03 May 2020	Deaths/1M Population 12 Dec 2021	Median age (yrs)	Overweight %	%Fully Vaccinated as on 12 Dec 2021
USA	204	2450	38.1	67.9	60.6
Spain	540	1889	42.5	61.6	79.6
Italy	475	2234	45.5	58.5	74.3
France	379	1838	41.4	59.5	71
UK	414	2140	40.5	63.7	69.47
Germany	81	1262	47.1	56.8	69.5
Brazil	35	2873	42.4	57.3	65.6
Sweden	265	1488	41.2	56.4	70.17
Belarus	10	557	40	59.4	30.5

Table 2. Deaths from Covid-19 in some Asian Countries

Country	Deaths/1M population 03 May 2020	Deaths/1M Population 12 Dec 2021	Median age (yrs)	Overweight %	% Fully Vaccinated as on 12 Dec 2021
India	1.0	340	27.9	19.7	36.37
Pakistan	2	127	23.8	28.4	25.41
Afghanistan	2	182	18.8	23	9.27
Sri Lanka	0.3	677	32.8	23.3	63.47
Bangladesh	1	177	26.7	20	25.31
Maldives	2	464	28.2	30.6	62.5
Nepal	Nil	386	24.1	21	29.9
Japan	3.86	146	48.4	24.6	77.8

Table 3. Deaths from Covid-19 in some African Countries

Country	Deaths/1M population 03 May 2020	Deaths/1M Population 12 Dec 2021	Median age (yrs)	Overweight %	% Fully Vaccinated as on 12 Dec 2021
Nigeria	0.4	14	18.4	28.9	1.9
Ethiopia	0.03	57	17.9	20.9	1.32
Egypt	4	200	23.9	63.5	14.41
DR Congo	0.4	12	28.1	25.3	0.18
Tanzania	0.3	12	17.7	26.0	1.51
South Africa	2	1492	27.1	53.8	29.36
Kenya	0.4	96	19.7	25.5	5.98
Uganda	Nil	68	15.8	22.4	2.87

What did we miss? Why we kept insisting on one size fits all? Obviously something was very different on the white and black side of the chess board. Let us look at the other pieces on the board. As will seem striking from the Tables, the Western countries have much higher median age and much higher levels of obesity compared to the Asian and African countries. Older age is associated with higher fatality from Covid-19. So is obesity, it compromises lung function and also is a surrogate marker for other co-morbidities such as hypertension and diabetes, conditions increasing bad outcome from Covid-19 infection. It seems that even a little higher prevalence of obesity increases mortality from Covid-19. Among African countries, Egypt and South Africa are having higher obesity rates and also higher mortality in Africa from Covid-19 albeit far lower than the Western countries. The experience of two countries, Japan and Brazil also offers some leads to which of the two factors, age or obesity, is greater risk for mortality from Covid-19. Japan has high median age, higher than most Western countries. However, this disadvantage is offset by lower rate of overweight compared to the West. Brazil on the other hand has younger population but higher proportion of overweight people. Japan, in spite of higher age has much lower deaths from Covid-19 compared to Brazil and most Western countries which indicates that obesity is a major risk factor of adverse outcome from Covid-19

Some have also suggested that past infections with other coronaviruses, likely in overcrowded living conditions may offer cross immunity against Covid-19 – this has to be confirmed by proper studies.

Eyeballing the data in the tables suggest that the percentage of population fully vaccinated also do not correlate with death rates from Covid-19 at the country level. This should be cause for concern as the world is single mindedly pursuing the target of universal mass vaccination at astronomical costs.

It is possible that factors like lower age of population, lower prevalence of overweight and past infections with other coronaviruses may be acting in combination (like weaker chess pieces) to trap the Covid-19 queen on the black side of the chess board, and vaccination like other blunt and often draconian measures implemented earlier may have very modest impact. A study done by researchers of Harvard University and published in the European Journal of Epidemiology is also sobering. This paper reports that there was no impact of mass vaccination on Covid-19 incidence across 68 countries and 2947 US counties.

The take home message is that the epidemiological approach should see all the factors and their combinations across different countries and regions to cope with the present and future pandemics.

9 789393 388698

Printed by Libri Plureos GmbH in Hamburg, Germany